SHINRIN YOKU

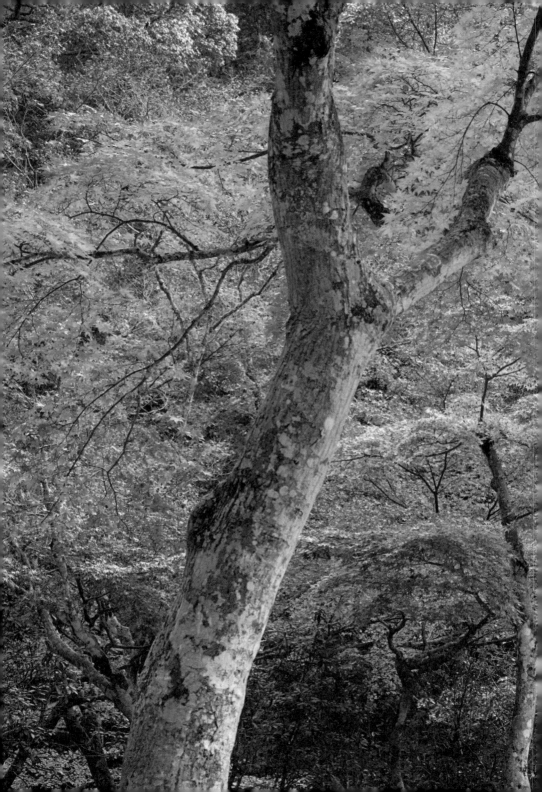

Yoshifumi Miyazaki

THE JAPANESE ART OF

shinrin
yoku

FOREST BATHING

Timber Press
PORTLAND, OREGON

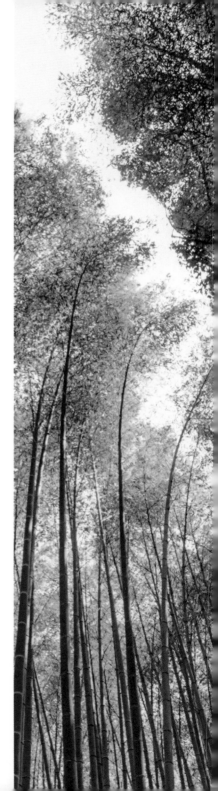

First published in Great Britain in 2018 by
Aster, a division of Octopus Publishing Group Ltd.
Text copyright © Yoshifumi Miyazaki 2018
Design & layout copyright © Octopus Publishing
Group Ltd. 2018

Published in the United States and Canada in
2018 by Timber Press, Inc.

The Haseltine Building
133 S.W. Second Avenue, Suite 450
Portland, Oregon 97204-3527
timberpress.com

ISBN 978-1-60469-879-4

A catalog record for this book is available
from the Library of Congress.

Picture Library Manager Jennifer Veall
Production Manager Caroline Alberti
Cover design Adrianna Sutton

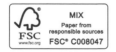

Contents

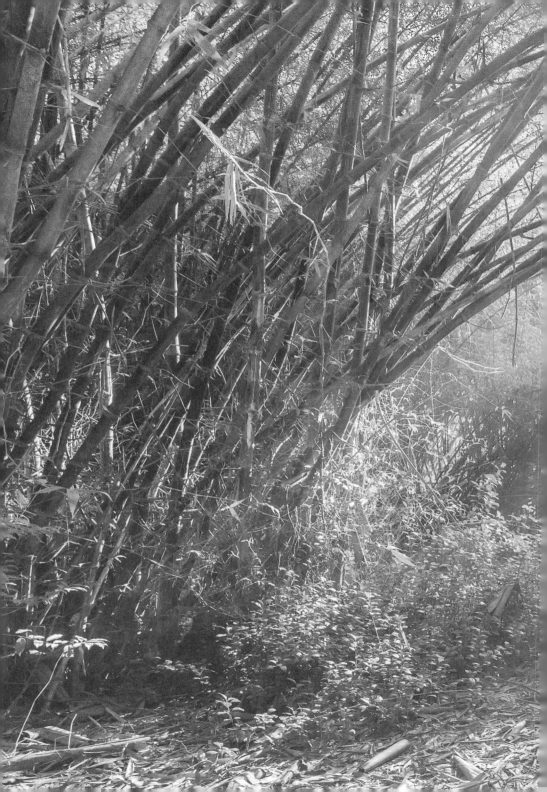

"Not knowing the
name of the tree,
I stood in the flood
of its sweet scent"

— MATSUO BASHŌ

Imagine taking a walk in the forest right now. You feel the earth and leaves under your feet, the snap of twigs. You listen to the birdsong and look up through the breaks in the canopy to the sky above, noticing how the light filters through to a point just further along the path.

You breathe in, deeply.

You smell the distinct forest aromas: moss, sap, earth and wood.

You take it all in.

Introduction

In Japan there is a notable preventative medicine that is being practised by increasing numbers of the population. Although it was borne out of intuition, this medicine is now being supported by a growing body of scientific research which endorses its many benefits.

The word *shinrin-yoku* was coined in 1982 by Tomohide Akiyama[1], Director of the Japanese Forestry Agency. It can be translated literally as "forest bathing" and is used in a similar way to "sun bathing" and "sea bathing". You don't literally take a bath, but you do bathe in the environment of the forest, using all your senses to experience nature up close.

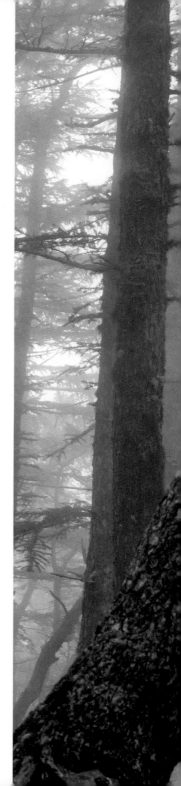

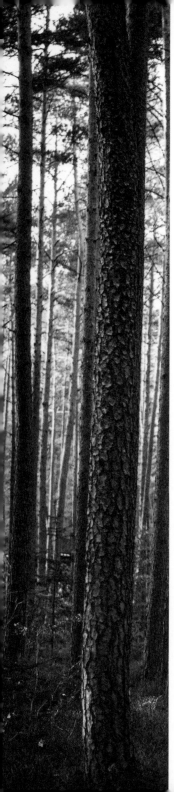

WHAT IS *SHINRIN-YOKU?*

Simply put, *shinrin-yoku* is the practice of walking slowly through the woods, in no hurry, for a morning, an afternoon or a day. When the phrase was first coined, the idea was more of a marketing exercise to attract people to the many beautiful forests of Japan, but since then myself and a number of other scientists in Japan and other countries around the world have begun to study the physiological and psychological effects of nature, and specifically forests, on human health and wellbeing. It is the understanding that somehow we feel better when we are surrounded by nature that has inspired this research.

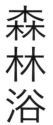

The Japanese characters for *shinrin-yoku*. The first character is a forest (three trees), the second a wood (two trees), and the third "bathe" (flowing water on the left, and a valley on the right).

In March 1990 I conducted the first experiments to study the physiological effects of *shinrin-yoku* on the Japanese island of Yakushima.[2~4] With the cooperation of NHK (Japan Broadcasting Corporation) we began our experiments to measure levels of the stress hormone cortisol in the saliva of subjects walking through a forest. But for around a decade afterward, little progress was made in the collection of scientific and physiological data. Since 2000, however, science has moved on and we now have new techniques to measure brain activity and autonomic nervous activity, both good indicators of the level of stress in the human body. These last 10–15 years, data has accumulated rapidly.

The findings have been extremely encouraging; it is clear that our bodies still recognize nature as our home, which is important to consider as increasing numbers of people are living in cities and urban environments each year.

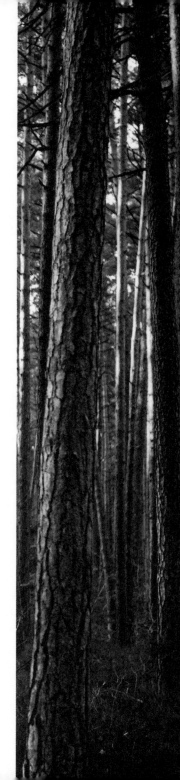

WHY DO WE NEED
SHINRIN-YOKU?

In recent years, stress-related diseases have become a social problem on a global scale. Without even realizing it, we are over-stimulated and stressed by today's man-made world, and that makes our bodies more susceptible to disease. It is not surprising that attention is turning to *shinrin-yoku* as an example of a natural and low-cost way to alleviate this problem.

It is around seven million years since our ancestors started evolving into the modern humans we are today.[5] During this process of evolution we have spent more than 99.99 per cent of our time living in a natural environment. Our bodies are adapted to nature.[6,7] *Shinrin-yoku* cannot treat disease, but it can have a preventative medical effect that makes falling ill less likely, and can help reduce the strain on health services worldwide that stress-related illnesses cause each year.

It is only over the last 10–15 years that enough data has accumulated to allow us to shape the practice of *shinrin-yoku* with science.[8–30] In 2003 I proposed the term "forest therapy" to describe *shinrin-yoku* supported by scientific evidence. What started as an intuitive-based therapy has become an evidence-based therapy, and can now be considered to be a preventative medicine.

There are currently more than 60 official forest therapy trails in Japan, designated for the practice of *shinrin-yoku* by the Forest Therapy Society. There is also a growing number of doctors who are certified in forest medicine.

MY BACKGROUND

I would like to explain how I came to be a forest therapy researcher, starting with my early life. I was born in 1954, and from my earliest memories I have always loved nature. When I was nine years old we moved to a house with a garden and I came into contact with soil for the first time. My father loved plants and I can remember helping him with jobs in the garden, such as replanting trees. I also remember wondering why my body felt so relaxed when I came into contact with soil, flowers and trees. When I did my university entrance exams I decided to study agriculture – I'm not completely sure why, but perhaps that question from my childhood still remained.

As a child I wasn't an able student. I was bottom of the class in the first year of elementary school and never achieved a score of more than 20 per cent in tests. Looking back, I don't think I understood the concept of test questions and answers, and didn't know what to write in the answer column. I was that kind of child.

Today, I am a professor at Chiba University. Yet when I applied to study at the same university all those years ago, I failed the entrance exams twice. I couldn't get into Chiba University as a student, but eventually I became a professor here. Things have worked our rather strangely.

Although I failed to get into Chiba University, I did eventually manage to secure a place to study at Tokyo University of Agriculture and Technology. However, I neglected my studies and spent all of my time playing sports and looking after my tropical fish. Because of that, I scraped through my exams with the minimum grades to achieve a pass. I made no effort to find a job and had no option other than to continue in education and progress to a masters course.

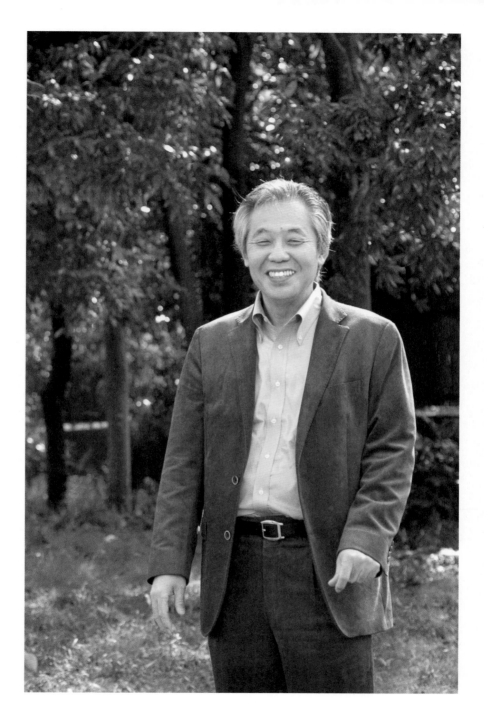

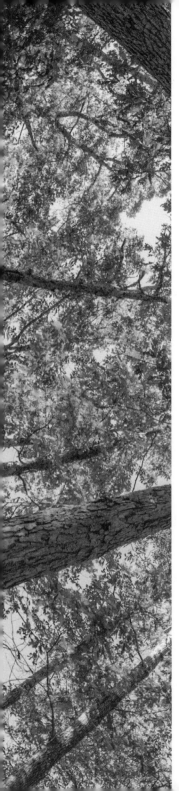

Until that point, the university only accepted ten students each year on its masters course, but that year the number was increased to twelve. I was the twelfth student, again only scraping through. I finished my masters course and once again I hadn't thought about looking for any work. However, a position suddenly appeared for an assistant professor in the Faculty of Medicine at the Tokyo Medical and Dental University. My professor at the time told me that he didn't know whether I could do it, but it would be a waste not to try.

I got the job and started on the winding road of my research career. As I didn't have any medical qualifications, I faced various difficulties working in a medical department, but at the same time I had the chance to learn about research techniques. The Tokyo Medical and Dental University has one of Japan's leading faculties of medicine, and my tutor was able to teach me the basic skills of research. I realized that I would need to get a PhD if I wanted to continue working as a researcher, so I gritted my teeth, achieved a PhD in medicine and spent a total of nine years working in the department.

In 1988, I was employed by Japan's Forestry and Forest Products Research Institute (FFPRI). This was the start of my *shinrin-yoku* research. At the institute we were free to choose our research topics, so I focused on forests, timber and relaxation. I wanted to find answers to a question that had interested me since childhood: "Why do we feel relaxed when we encounter nature?" However, as I was still very young I couldn't get the research funds I needed.

Luckily, I received a request from NHK, Japan's national broadcasting company, who wanted me to work on a programme about Yakushima, an island in Japan known for its cedar forests. This stroke of good fortune led to the world's first physiological experiments on *shinrin-yoku*: research into the effects of Yakushima cedar on stress hormones in the human body.

This work led, in 2004, to a large research budget from the Japanese government and the start of proper forest therapy research. After spending 19 years as a researcher at the FFPRI, I moved to the Center for Environment, Health and Field Sciences at Chiba University.

I had worked in the Faculty of Agriculture, as an assistant professor in the Faculty of Medicine, as a team leader at the FFPRI, then finally became a professor at the university. My research career has bridged the fields of environmental protection, medicine, forestry and health science, and has had plenty of twists and turns. But all the different fields of research have greatly benefitted the forest therapy research I am doing now, and have shaped the way I work.

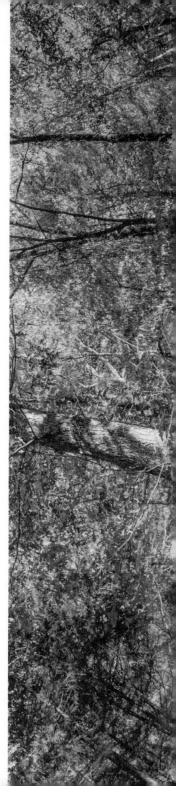

"The tree which moves some to tears of joy is in the eyes of others only a green thing that stands in the way. Some see Nature all ridicule and deformity, and some scarce see Nature at all. But to the eyes of the man of imagination, Nature is Imagination itself."

— WILLIAM BLAKE

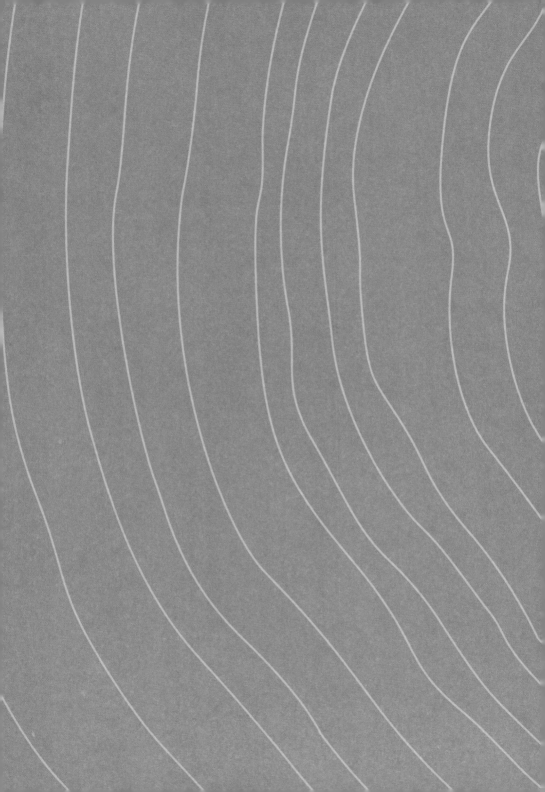

—

CHAPTER 1

The Concept of Nature Therapy

自然セラピーの概念

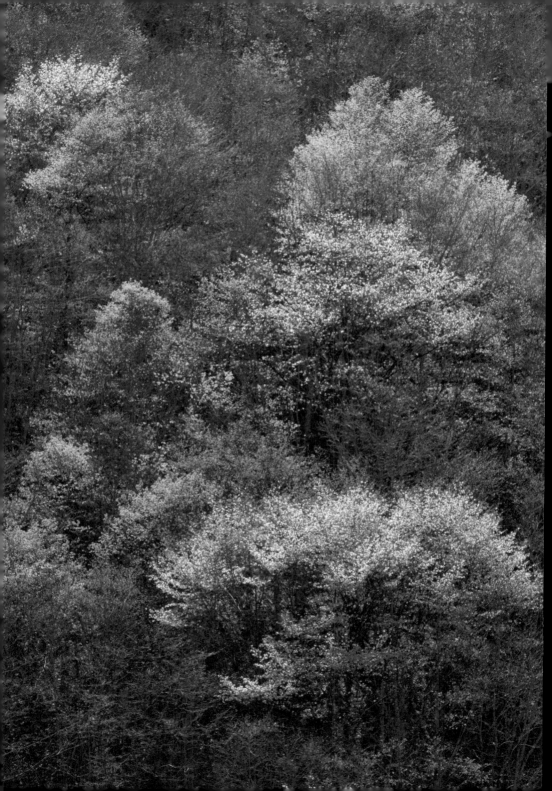

Stress and stress-related diseases have become a burden to modern society and attention is turning to the forests and the natural world, an environment familiar to us for millions of years, to offer a solution. As we saw in the introduction, nature therapies are a new concept that use a preventative approach to lower stress levels, improve quality of life and potentially reduce the cost and strain on health services that stress-related illnesses cause.

Intuitively, we understand that the natural world makes us feel relaxed. The idea behind nature therapy is to clarify those effects with science, and to use them as a preventative medicine to improve wellbeing in our modern world. Nature therapy is natural, non-invasive and harnesses a quality our bodies already possess: their adaptation to nature.

It is not just forests that can have a beneficial effect on our wellbeing. Other natural stimuli, such as parks, flowers, bonsai and even pieces of wood have been shown to reduce stress, making these effects attainable for all of us, even city-dwellers.

The aims of nature therapy

Our bodies have become adapted to nature over millions of years of evolution. Even though we may struggle to realize it, living in our modern society puts us in a permanent condition of stress. That is why having contact with nature can help us enter a state of physiological relaxation, as well as bring us closer to our original natural state as humans.

The basic concept[6,7] behind nature therapy is to increase physiological relaxation and act as a preventative medicine by improving the body's natural resistance to disease, which is suppressed under conditions of stress.

What's more, nature therapy has a physiological adjustment effect,[8] which means that it has a different effect on different individuals. At first we thought that there were errors in the way the data was collected but we have since found that the different results experienced by different people are in fact real. A good example is blood pressure. We found that forest therapy reduces blood pressure in those individuals who start with high blood pressure, while it increases blood pressure in those individuals who start with low blood pressure. This effect makes the therapy especially valuable as it adjusts to the individual, but we need to do more research to find out how and why this happens.

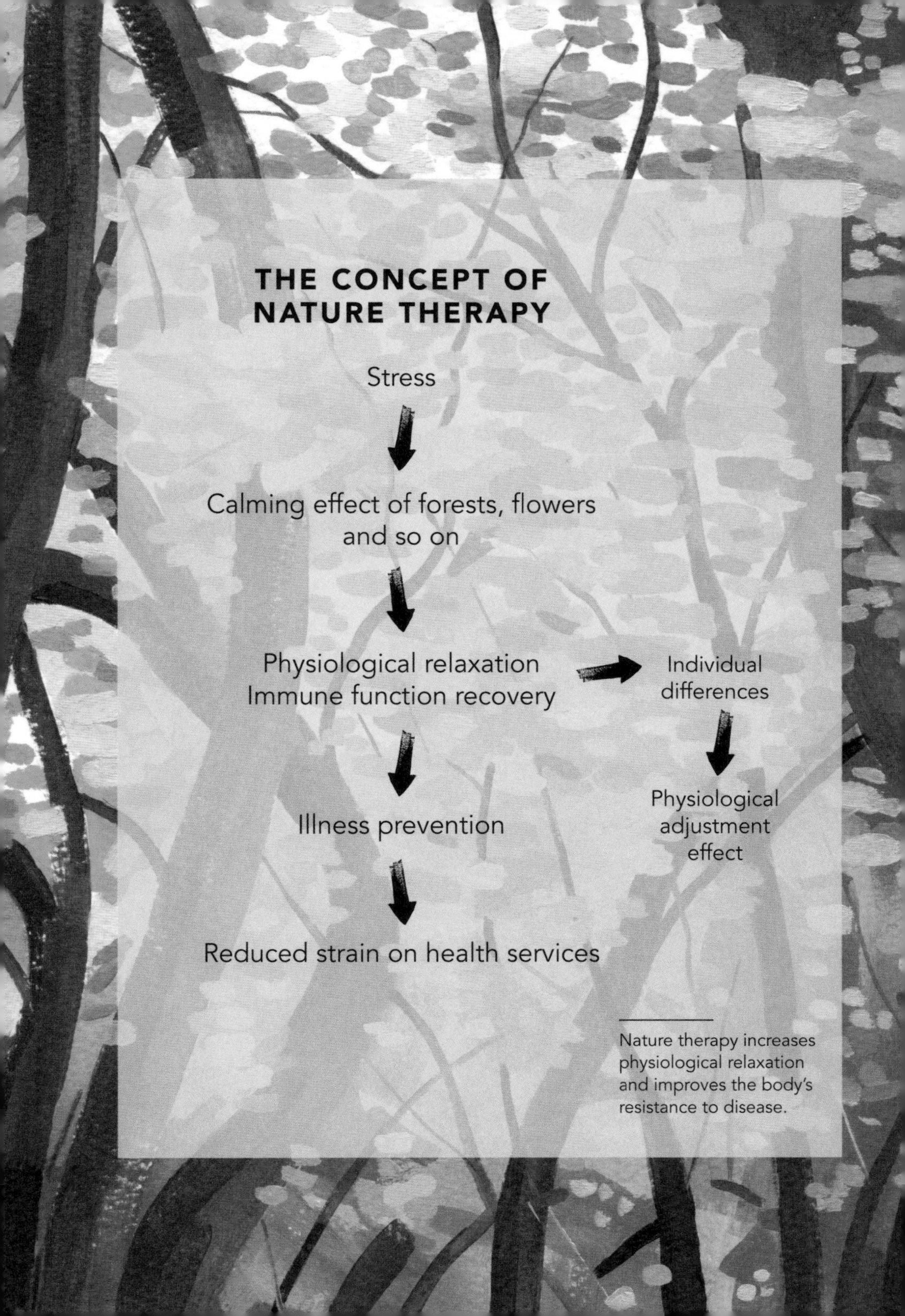

THE CONCEPT OF
NATURE THERAPY

Stress

↓

Calming effect of forests, flowers
and so on

↓

Physiological relaxation   →   Individual
Immune function recovery   differences

↓   ↓

Illness prevention   Physiological
                                   adjustment
↓   effect

Reduced strain on health services

Nature therapy increases
physiological relaxation
and improves the body's
resistance to disease.

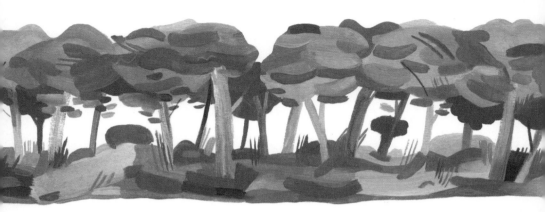

Back to Nature theory

Around seven million years have passed since our ancestors started down the path that has led to the humans we are today.[5] As it is only two or three hundred years since the Industrial Revolution, when vast numbers of us moved to urban surroundings, we can say that humans have spent over 99.99 per cent of their time in a natural environment.

In 1800, only 3 per cent of the world's population lived in urban areas. By 1900, this figure was close to 14 per cent and in 2016 this reached 54 per cent. The United Nations Population Division predicts that by 2050, this figure will reach 66 per cent.

But genes cannot change over just a few hundred years, so we live in our modern society with bodies that are still adapted to the natural environment.

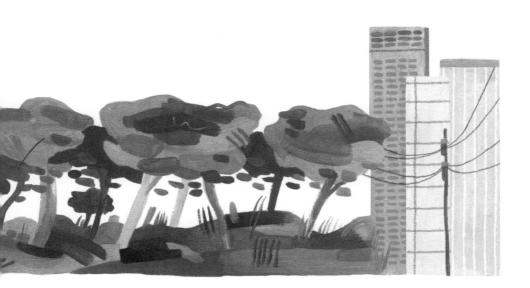

Inevitably, we are in a state of constant stress and the recent rapid spread of computer technology has made this state of stress even worse. In 1984, the American clinical psychologist Craig Brod came up with the term "technostress". In the three decades since, our world has become even more reliant on technology and even further removed from nature.

My own academic mentor, the physiological anthropologist Masahiko Sato, described in one of his works how cities appeared only very recently in human history,[31] how all our physiological functions evolved in a natural environment, and how those functions were made for a natural environment. When we come into contact with nature such as forests, parks and flowers, we feel relaxed. That is because our bodies (including our genes) were made to be adapted to nature. Inspired by the New Zealand researchers Mary Ann O'Grady and Lonny Meinecke,[32] I call this Back to Nature theory.

Humans have spent over 99.99 per cent of their time throughout history in a natural environment. This explains why humans have become adapted to nature.

Nature therapy and wellbeing

There is an ever-growing interest in health and wellbeing around the world. Being "healthy" no longer means only freedom from disease as it once did. In my own understanding, being healthy is a state in which the individual can fully exhibit the abilities he or she has. Or, in other words, the state of being healthy is relative to the individual rather than being absolute. Being healthy is also a process – it is the way in which we live.

URBANIZATION

According to a 2014 UN report, 54 per cent of the world's population lives in urban areas, a proportion that is expected to increase to 66 per cent by 2050. Sustainable urbanization is therefore crucial to successful development, and this includes considering the health and wellbeing of city-dwellers.

Cities are not inherently bad for us, but our bodies need nature in order to regulate and feel more comfortable. This was our understanding, but if we were to make forest therapy acknowledged as a preventative medicine available to all, we needed to prove how our physiology responds to different habitats.

LIVING IN THE 21ST CENTURY

There isn't really a word for "stress" in Japanese, so we often use the English term "stress" instead. This isn't to say we don't experience stress in Japan. In recent decades there has been an increase in pressure to work long hours, get good grades in education and be successful in life.

Throughout the world, we are living in societies characterized by urbanization, yet our physiological functions are still adapted to nature. Because of this, the sympathetic nervous system is in a constant state of over-stimulation and stress levels are often too high. Poor sleep and the shortage of opportunities to relax contribute to the lack of healthy regulation in the nervous system.

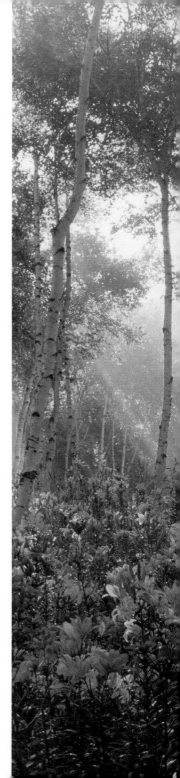

FIGHT OR FLIGHT

Sympathetic nervous system

The sympathetic nervous system is mobilized by the fight-or-flight response. The fight-or-flight response is an acute stress response to a stressor. Under stress, our body has a fifth gear, powered by adrenalin. When something in our environment triggers our brain's alarm system, our body will automatically go into survival mode, shutting down part of our conscious brain to allow our physical instincts to take over, in other words so that we can either fight or take flight.

The problem with 21st-century living is that our stress response system isn't only triggered by physically dangerous situations but also by emotionally dangerous situations. The crowd on the commuter train, the driver who takes the parking space you wanted, the employer who isn't happy with your report. There is also the constant stimulation provided by technology ("technostress"), which prevents people from taking enough time to relax and allow the body and mind to rest fully.

Therefore, modern life is full of stimuli that can trigger the sympathetic nervous system. And when the body remains in this activated state for too long, a state of hyper-arousal can occur.

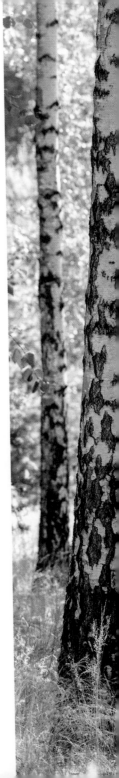

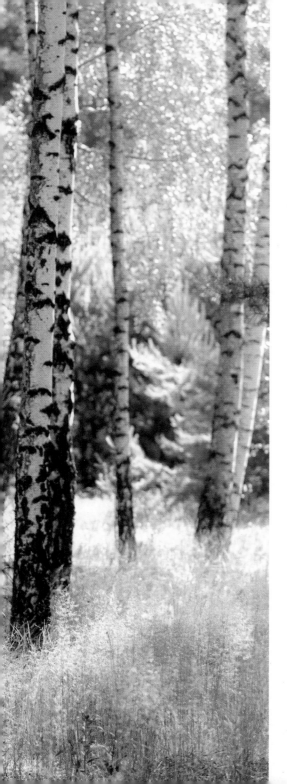

REST AND DIGEST

Parasympathetic nervous system

On the other hand, the other part of the autonomic nervous system, the parasympathetic nervous system, regulates the body, allowing it to rest and digest. It is responsible for restoring the body to a state of calm and in this state it performs various tasks of repair.

However, when the human body experiences too much chronic stress over too long a period of time, the parasympathetic nervous system might collapse.

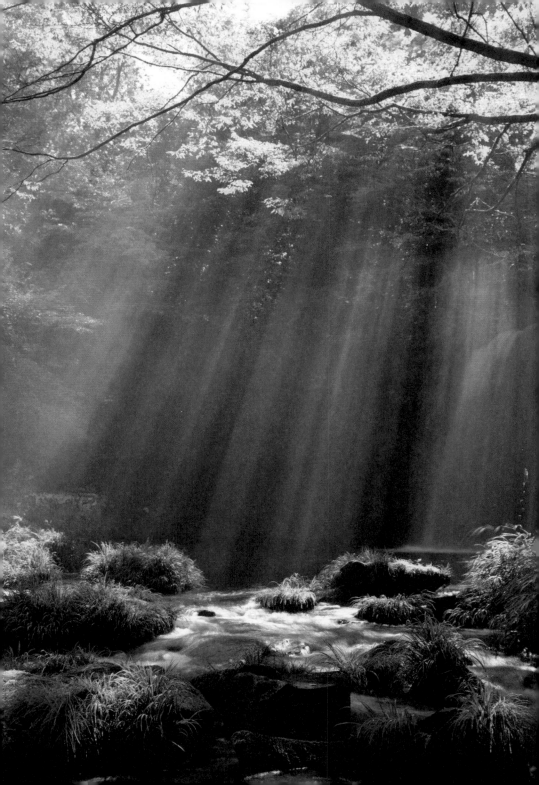

NATURE AND THE NERVOUS SYSTEM

Regulating the nervous system is exactly where nature therapies come in. When in a natural environment, stress is reduced and people report a feeling of relaxation. They also report feelings of being energized and refreshed. This simple act helps to regulate the nervous system, promoting a healthier balance between activation and relaxation, which in my view is a fundamental marker of wellbeing. In this way, illness can be prevented and a healthy way of living is maintained.

Stress-related illnesses

The following illnesses and conditions have been shown to be related to chronic stress:

- The common cold
- Back, neck and shoulder pain
- Slower healing
- Weight gain and loss
- Sleep dysfunction
- Depression
- Dysautonomia
- Irritable bowel syndrome
- Ulcers and stomach problems
- Heart disease
- Cancer risk

Nature as medicine

Although the simple act of walking in a forest might not seem extraordinary, the benefits that people experience during and after a session of forest therapy really are.

THE BENEFITS OF *SHINRIN-YOKU*

We have measured the following direct benefits of forest therapy:

· Improvement of weakened immunity, with an increase in the count of natural killer (NK) cells, which are known to fight tumours and infection

· Increased relaxation of the body due to increased activity in the parasympathetic nervous system

· Reduced stress of the body due to a reduction in sympathetic nervous system activity

· Reduction in blood pressure after only 15 minutes of forest therapy

· Reduced feelings of stress and a general sense of wellbeing

· Reduction in blood pressure after 1 day of forest therapy, which lasts up to 5 days after therapy

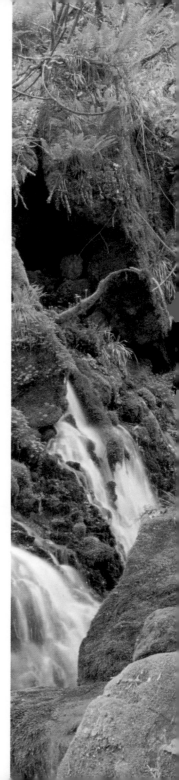

The restorative power of nature

Scientists in Pennsylvania showed that even the view from your window can have a beneficial effect. They studied patients who were recovering in hospital after they had had an operation to remove their gall bladders. Some patients were assigned a room with a window that looked out on a brick wall, others had a room with a view of a natural scene. They found that the patients with a view of nature recovered more quickly, were able to leave hospital sooner and requested fewer painkillers during their stay.[33]

Why does nature reduce stress?

Most of us would agree that being surrounded by nature makes us feel "comfortable", and this is the reason we experience a reduction in stress levels. I believe it is important to explore what we mean by "comfort", and as there isn't yet a recognized definition, I'd like to offer one here.

SYNCHRONIZATION OF RHYTHM

My conception of comfort is "a situation where human and natural rhythms are synchronized". When we are in a particular environment and we feel that our own rhythms synchronize with the rhythms of that environment, we feel comfortable. If during a lecture the audience makes attentive noises and is interested, the speech will be lively. But if they glance around or nod off, the speech will falter. It is the same at a concert.

I believe that we can discuss comfort from the perspective of whether people are synchronized with their environment, or not. Of course, this environment includes not just people, but also animals and plants, as well as films, music and other inanimate things.

Most of us have day-to-day experience of how contact with plants and flowers automatically makes us feel relaxed. For example, in the corner of this room as I write are two plants, a papaya plant and an avocado plant which I grew from seeds after eating the fruit. The other day I picked a delicious ripe papaya and ate it. When I am tired by writing, I can feel relaxation just by glancing at the plant. I can feel synchronization from even this small example of nature, a potted plant. This must surely be connected to how, over the seven million years of human evolution, we have lived amid nature and our bodies have adapted to that nature.

PASSIVE COMFORT VS ACTIVE COMFORT

In 1961, the World Health Organization characterized a lifestyle as having four layers: comfort, efficiency, health and safety. Masao Inui divided comfort into two types, naming them "passive comfort" and "active comfort".[34] Based on Inui's ideas, I have also differentiated between passive and active comfort (see diagram, opposite).

Passive comfort is based on so-called "deprivation needs", such as thermal regulation, and is a negative need that aims to eliminate discomfort. As a result, we can easily agree on what constitutes passive comfort because personal ideas and feelings are not involved. We need to stay warm, for example. On the other hand, active comfort, which is related to our sense of wellbeing, aims to gain something extra and we might all define this in a different way, resulting in large differences between individuals.

When I was at school some 50 years ago, the environment around me was not what we could call "comfortable". Atmospheric pollution was a problem, while living spaces were too cold during the winter and too hot during the summer. There really was a need for passive comfort back then.

By the start of the 1990s, however, those problems had been solved and society's interest had shifted to active comfort provided by the five senses. Society wants to know more about what active comfort or "wellbeing" is, but the topic is difficult to discuss academically.

PASSIVE COMFORT

Elimination of discomfort;
Little individual difference

ACTIVE COMFORT

Gain of something extra;
Great individual difference

Meeting
basic needs

Stimulation of
the five senses

Passive comfort relates to
our basic needs, such as
the need to stay warm.
Active comfort relates to
our sense of wellbeing.

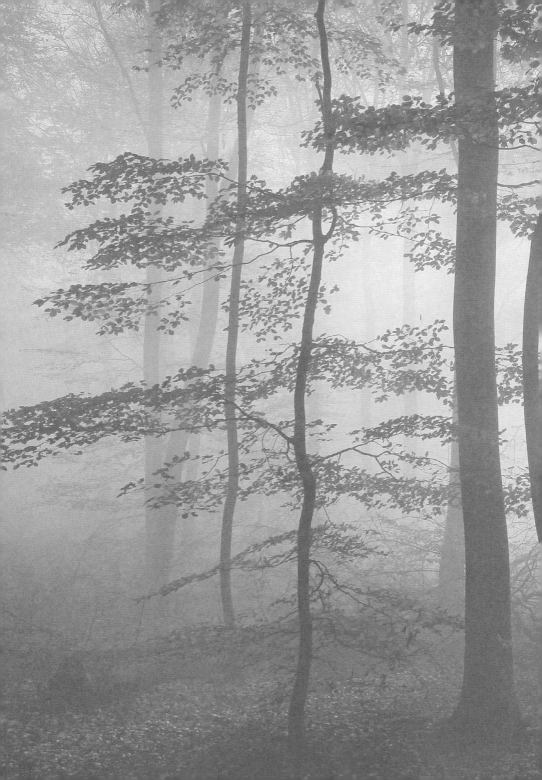

"I frequently tramped eight or ten miles through the deepest snow to keep an appointment with a beech tree, or a yellow birch, or an old acquaintance among the pines."

— HENRY DAVID THOREAU

—

CHAPTER 2

Japan's Relationship with Nature

日本人と自然の関係

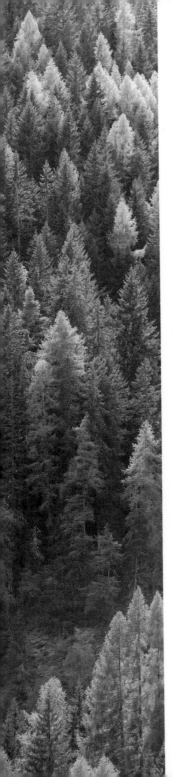

One New Year's Day in Japan, a discussion took place on television between the flower arranger Toshiro Kawase and the biologist Toshitaka Hidaka (my biology teacher at university). During the discussion, Kawase mentioned the difference between the Japanese approach to flower arranging and the European approach to flower arranging. In the Japanese tradition, the arranger offers thanks to the flowers once they have been arranged, by performing a bow. This custom does not exist in European flower arranging and Kawase said that this bow of thanks given to the arranged flowers in Japan indicates equality between the person and the flowers.

In reply, Hidaka recalled how he had once praised a flower arrangement in a French home. When he was asked what he liked about it, he did not know how to explain his feelings. He felt the appeal of the flower arrangement as a whole, including his own personal relationship with the flowers, so he struggled to analyze it when asked.

Hidaka felt that this showed the special way Japanese people view nature. The Japanese do not see people as having a special place above nature; rather, people and the natural world exist as equals. Personally, I was fascinated at how they expressed the same thoughts about the relationship between people and nature, despite coming from two completely different fields – one a scientist, the other a flower arranger.

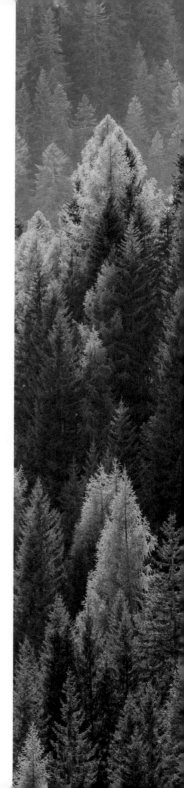

Nature in Japanese culture

There is a similar sentiment in a book by the Japanese writer Isamu Kurita called *A Flower Journey*.[35] He notes that, "In the West people look at flowers. In Asia, they live with them." This idea of a close bond between Japanese people and nature is not new. In many ancient poems, like those by Ki no Tsurayuki and Ono no Komachi written around 1,000 years ago, the lives and appearances of the poets are identified with those of the flowers.

Masao Watanabe, an Emeritus Professor at the University of Tokyo, expressed his thoughts on how Japanese people see nature in a 1974 edition of *Science*.[36] "According to the Christian religion, which has been followed in Western society, all in heaven and earth is the creation of God. Within that, Man alone is a special creation and a sharp line is drawn between Man and the rest of creation," he wrote. "We might say that Man's, and only Man's, place as a special creation above the rest of creation lies at the root of the West's view of nature. Also, in the West Man stands opposed to nature, but in Japan Man is part of nature."[37]

In the same essay, Haruhiko Morinaga looks at the issue from the perspective of Western absolutism vs Eastern relativity, and uses the following example to illustrate these deep cultural differences.[38] Someone asks: "A whale is not a fish, is it?" A Japanese person would reply, "Yes, of course, it is not a fish," to agree with the speaker. A person from the West, however, would simply answer "No, it is not a fish." The Westerner's answer is a simple statement of fact, while the Japanese person's answer is relative to the question. This Western absolutism and Eastern relativity may also apply to the relationship Japanese people have with nature.

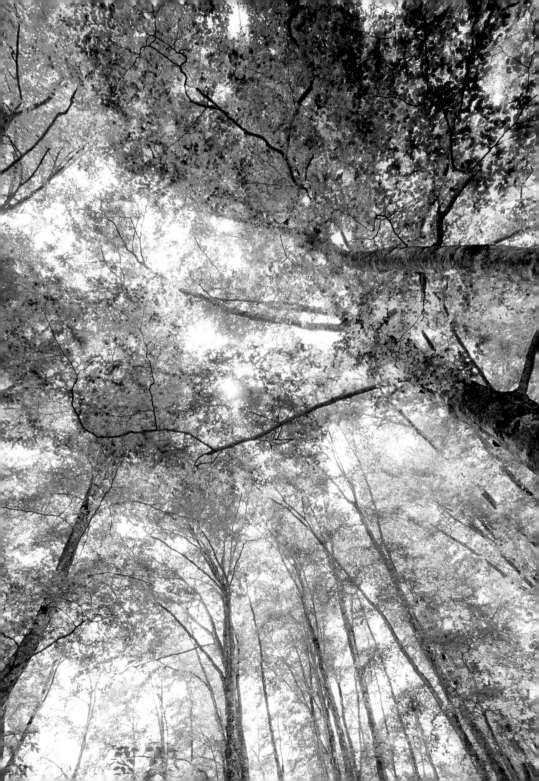

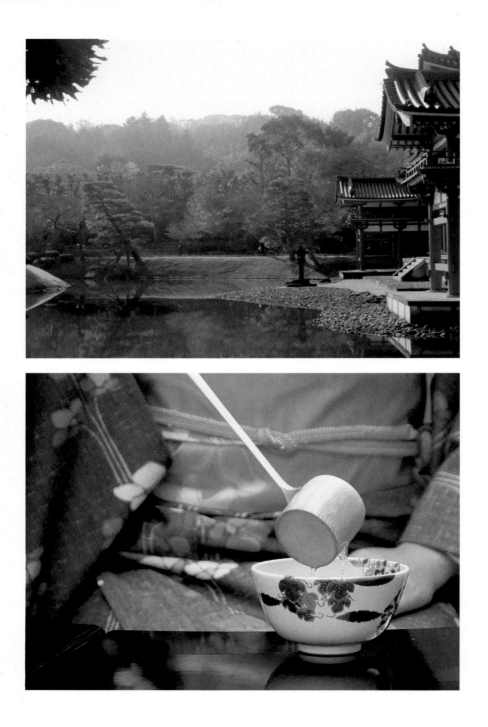

The Japanese aesthetic

Many commentators on Japanese culture observe the relationship between Japanese people and nature as part of the "Japanese aesthetic", a set of philosophical ideas that link Japanese art and life. One common thread is an appreciation of beauty that is imperfect and impermanent, which for many poets and artists is embodied by nature.

In the oldest known anthologies of Japanese poems, emotions were often expressed in terms of nature. In his preface to the *Kokinshu* poetry anthology, the Japanese author and poet Ki no Tsurayuki explains, "Japanese poetry has the hearts of men for its seeds, which grow into numerous leaves of words. People, as they experience various events in life, speak out their hearts in terms of what they see and hear."

There are also classic symbols that link nature with emotions; falling cherry blossoms are associated with sorrow, and an autumn evening is often used to express loneliness.

In modern Japan, these ideas are still in use, particularly in architecture, which is designed to be in harmony with the natural surroundings, garden design, crafts and product design.

"In spring it is the dawn that is most beautiful... In summer the nights. Not only when the moon shines, but on dark nights too, as the fireflies flit to and fro, and even when it rains, how beautiful it is!"

—SEI SHONAGON

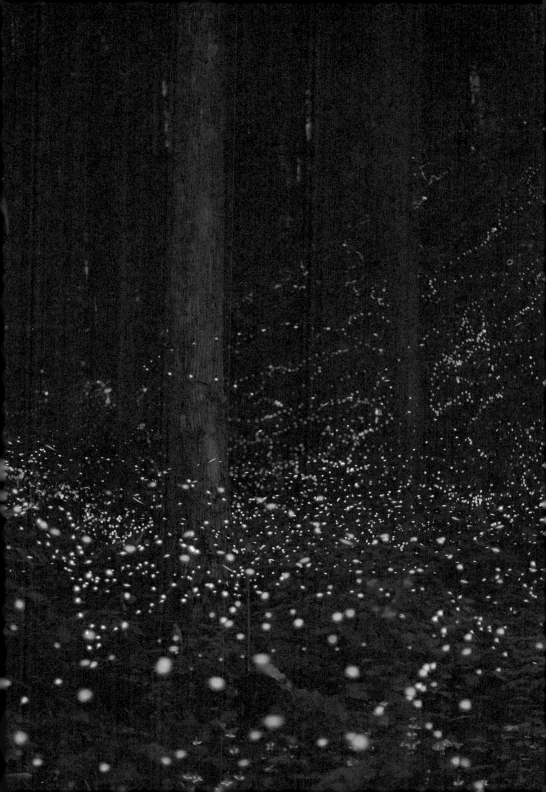

The geography of Japan

The Japanese archipelago is long and thin, extending about 3,000km (1,860 miles) from north to south. The climate and geography provide conditions for a wide range of tree species, varying from the mangrove swamps in the south of the country, up through deciduous broadleaves such as Japanese beech in the middle of the country, and then to conifers in the north.

The flora of Japan is marked by a large variety of species: around 5,560 plant species are native to Japan and this large number of plants reflects the diversity of climate that characterizes the Japanese archipelago.

There are over 249,850 square km (96,470 square miles) of forest in the country, covering 69 per cent of the total area of Japan. Of the industrialized nations of the world, Sweden and Finland are the only countries to have similarly high densities of forest, yet Japan is also one of the most densely populated countries on earth.

There are five climate zones with differing types of fauna and trees in each. *Matsu* and *sugi*, Japanese pine and cedar, respectively, are common throughout Japan – even in warm southern regions – and are very familiar to the Japanese people. There are three main kinds of natural forests in Japan:

· **Coniferous forest** of spruce and fir in alpine zones and eastern and northern Hokkaido
· **Deciduous forest** with oaks and beeches, in central Honshu and southern Hokkaido
· **Broadleaf evergreen forest** with laurel and chiquapin in western Honshu, Shikoku and Kyushu

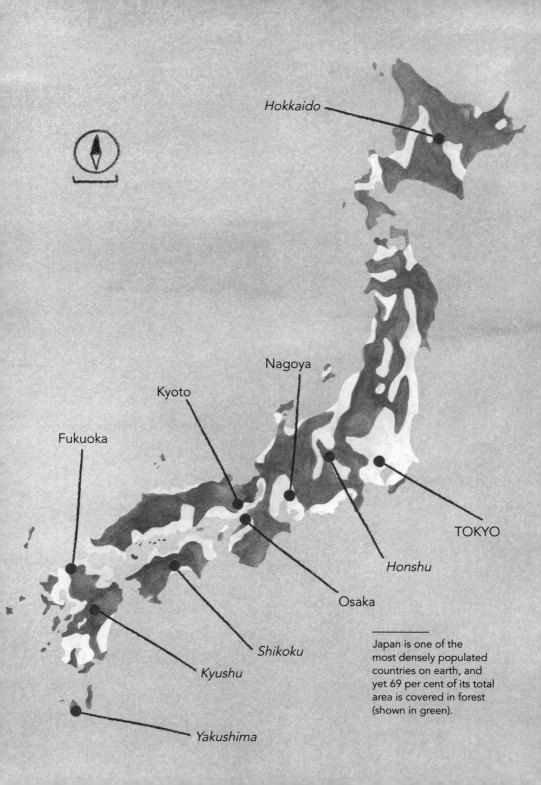

Hokkaido

Nagoya

Kyoto

Fukuoka

TOKYO

Honshu

Osaka

Shikoku

Kyushu

Japan is one of the
most densely populated
countries on earth, and
yet 69 per cent of its total
area is covered in forest
(shown in green).

Yakushima

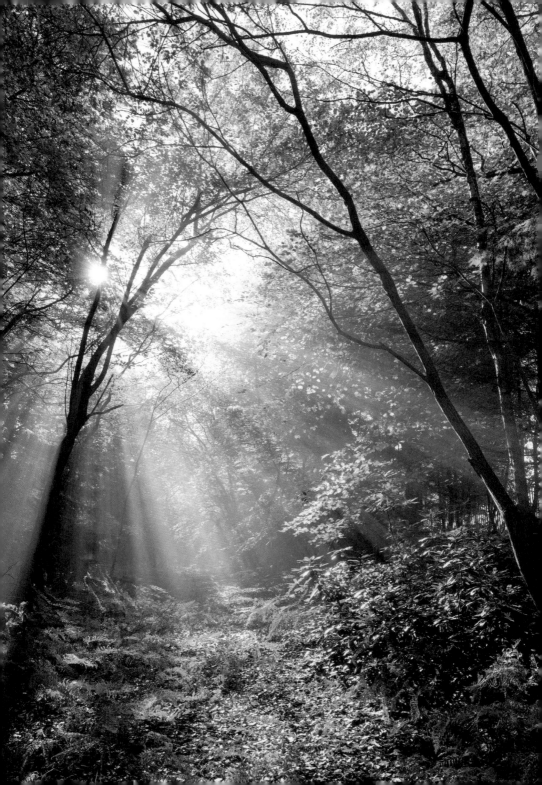

THE SIGNIFICANCE OF TREES IN JAPAN

Perhaps because such a large part of the country is populated by forest, trees are particularly revered in Japan, and exemplify the relationship of "man in harmony with nature". Their names alone show this special affinity. Pine trees (*Pinus thunbergii* and *Pinus densiflora*) are called *matsu*, which means "waiting for a god's soul to descend from heaven", while the name of the *ogatama-noki* tree (*Michelia compressa*) can be translated as "inviting soul". People believed that the tree had a special power to invite the soul of a god, so they used to plant it at the gate of a shrine.

CEDAR Large, old trees, such as Japanese cedar (*Cryptomeria japonica*), have a special significance as landmarks in Japan. They are revered for their stature and unique shape, for their record of climatic history in their annual rings, as examples of species that suit a particular environment, and as a guide to ecological rehabilitation of the surrounding area. It is believed that deities use these trees as landmarks when visiting on festival days.

Recently the Japanese have recognized the importance of these large trees, and attempts are being made to conserve them. There are even special doctors who can care for old weak trees. Growing at an altitude of 1,000m (3,280ft) on Yakushima Island, some giant Japanese cedars grow to heights of about 30m (100ft) and are over 2,000 years old. Small shrines are set on the trunks of these trees to reflect their spiritual significance.

KADOMATSU The tradition of decorating doorways at New Year with pine branches called *kadomatsu* (which literally means "gate pine") is still popular today and originally came from the belief that this was a way to welcome the gods to your home.

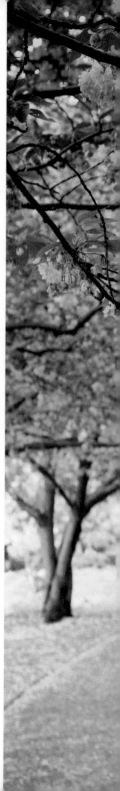

BAMBOO Bamboo (*Phyllostachys bambusoides*) often designates holy places. For example, when planting a tall bamboo called "the holy tree" on a paddy field, farmers customarily prayed to a god for a good rice harvest. Bamboo is revered for its rapid growth and symbolizes the mystery of strong life.

CHERRY BLOSSOM The centuries-old tradition of *hanami* (cherry blossom-viewing) is as popular today as it ever was. Many people flock to see the short-lived spectacle. The meaning of cherry blossom in Japan runs deep, making the country's national flower a cultural icon. Cherry blossom is revered not just for its overwhelming beauty, but for its enduring expression of life, death and renewal. Linked to the Buddhist themes of mortality, mindfulness and living in the present, cherry blossom is a timeless metaphor for human existence. The display of blossom is powerful, glorious and intoxicating, but tragically short-lived – a reminder that our lives, too, are fleeting but beautiful. This floral imagery permeates Japanese paintings, film and poetry.

BONSAI The art of growing miniature trees in pots was introduced to Japan in the 7th century. Like most Japanese art forms, bonsai is a complicated yet subtle process in which the desired effect arises from the simplicity of the aesthetic, the product of painstaking hard work and patience. Bonsai is governed by a set of aesthetic guidelines that range from an aversion to symmetry to a desire to recreate the proportions of a fully grown tree.

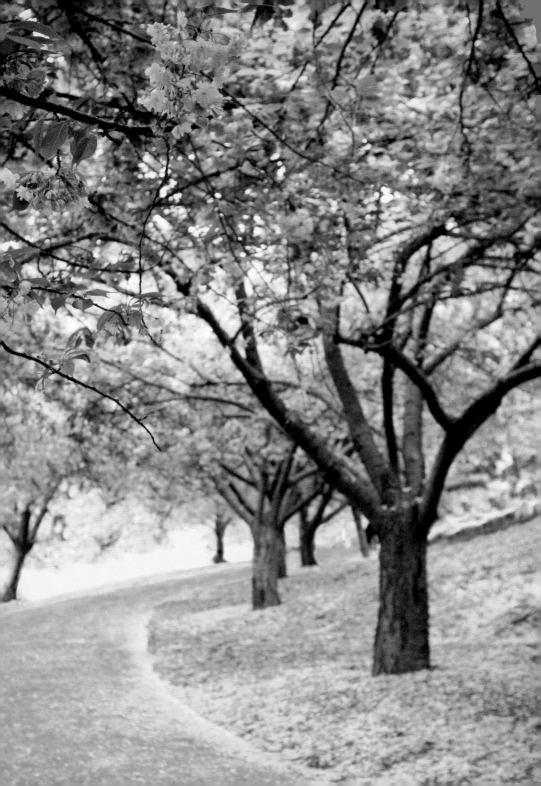

The study of nature therapy in Japan

It's no surprise, given the country's close bond with the natural world, in particular its forests and trees, that Japan is a leading player in research into nature therapies. Much of this work is backed by the Japanese government, which recognizes the need to reduce stress caused by the urban, artificial environment in which many Japanese people live. And why not look close to home for a solution? As we have seen, Japan is endowed with beautiful forests and wonderful natural spaces.

In 2004, we were able to acquire a large research budget of about 270 million yen (about 2.5 million dollars) for nature therapy research from the government, and an additional 200 million yen from the government's supplementary budget. With this funding we were able to build a climate-controlled test room and rapidly move our research forward.

During the last 15 years or so, Japanese manufacturers of physiological measuring devices have responded by developing the world's most advanced equipment to measure brain activity and autonomic nervous activity. This has contributed greatly to the progress of our research in the field of nature therapy in Japan.

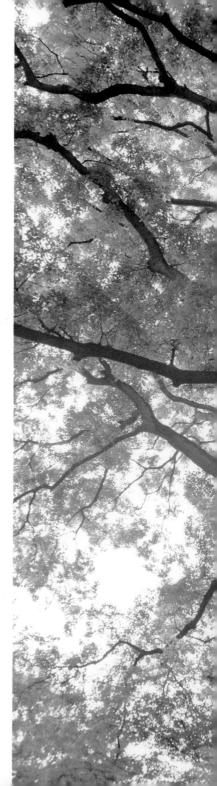

OUR RESEARCH SO FAR

Japan has amassed an impressive body of physiological data on not just *shinrin-yoku*, but also on other nature therapies such as park therapy,[39-44] wood therapy[45-54] and flower/bonsai therapy.[55-72]

The therapeutic value of the natural world is clear to see. In 1992, I conducted the first wood therapy experiments[45] and since then the results have been consistent. Simply by smelling or touching pieces of pine, oak or Japanese cypress wood, subjects experienced a calming of prefrontal brain activity, a reduction in sympathetic nerve activity and a rise in parasympathetic nerve activity (see pages 172-3) – all of which amounts to a reduction in stress.

Our research into park therapy and flower/bonsai therapy started in 2007. So far, we have conducted experiments to explore the benefits of walking in the park and while viewing roses, pansies, *Dracaena* and Japanese cypress bonsai. Other experiments have looked into the benefits of smelling roses and oranges, and also activities such as replanting ornamental plants. As with other nature therapies, we found clear evidence that these activities have a relaxing effect on the body (see pages 162-71).

"Mountains are not esteemed because they are high, but because they have trees"

— JAPANESE PROVERB

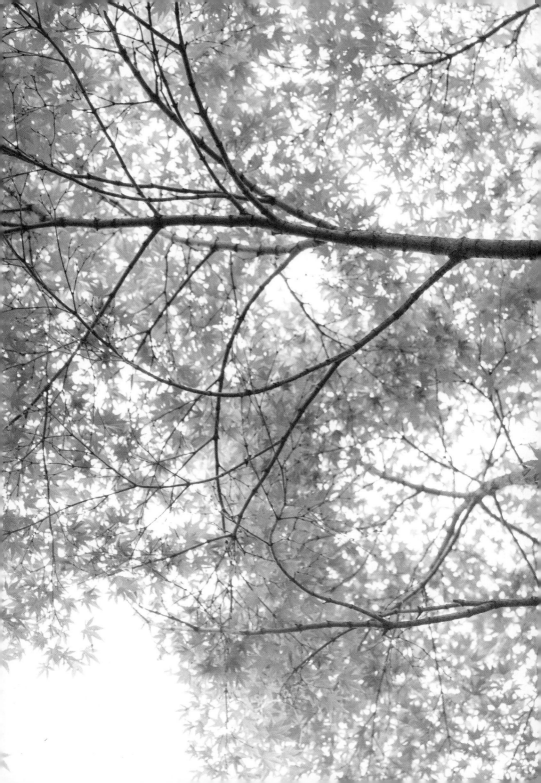

—

CHAPTER 3

The Practice
of *Shinrin-yoku*

森林浴の実践

What happens during a forest therapy session?
Over the following pages I will describe some of the
activities that take place at forest therapy bases in Japan.
Some of these may resonate with you as an individual.
Perhaps you would like to find a spot in a nearby forest
where you can meditate or practise yoga. Is there a
stream or lake in local woodland that you find relaxing?
Or maybe you would like to take a picnic along with
you on a forest walk to sit and enjoy halfway through?
You may notice the change of seasons more when
immersed in nature, or simply feel encouraged to take
in the sights and sounds of the trees around you.

Forest therapy activities

Many forest therapy programmes focus solely on walking and
seated viewing in forests. However, some of the more forward-
thinking forest therapy bases, like those mentioned on pages
74–7, offer a unique range of activities, all ingenious variations
on traditional forest therapy.

The purpose of forest therapy is to calm overstimulation from
artificial and urban environments and promote relaxation.
With this in mind, some of the more obvious activities include
meditation, yoga, stretching and hammock time. Some bases use
their physical surroundings to great effect and offer direct contact
with trees, waterfalls, night skies and snow-covered mountains
to offer relaxation effects. Others focus on the beauty of Japan
through the seasons, taking participants to enjoy cherry blossom,

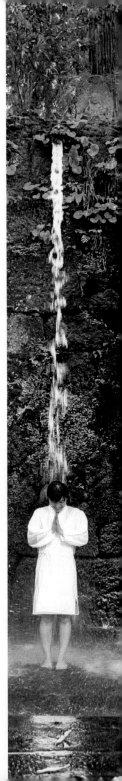

flowers and autumn foliage, or quintessentially Japanese features such as terraced rice fields, tea picking and hot springs. Some bases are even developing programmes to include music concerts, aroma workshops, horse riding, dog therapy and courses for children, involving catching fish and other activities.

Meditation and yoga

Our research has shown that simply sitting and enjoying the view in a forest offers physiological relaxation, but so far there has been no research on the relaxation effects of practising meditation and yoga in forests. We hope to contribute to further improvement of forest therapy programmes by investigating those effects, but so far these programmes have proved popular.

Hammock time

Another popular activity is hammock time, where participants lie in a hammock to take in the view of the forest. Lying down among trees is not something we do very often, so we expect this novel activity might have a major physiological relaxation effect. We are waiting for further research to prove this.

Water

Japan has many beautiful waterfalls and many bases include them in their forest therapy programmes. Japanese people particularly enjoy the practice of *takigyo*, seated meditation under a waterfall, which is offered at Kamiichi Town forest therapy base. The forest therapy programme in Ueno Village includes a unique course of supine rest in front of a waterfall. Yamakita Town and Yoshino Town

include stretching by a waterfall as one of their forest therapy activities, and the clear air and auditory stimulation of the waterfall are great attractions and add to the relaxation benefits.

Hot springs can also be found at many forest therapy bases, and participants are invited to take part in a walking course near the hot springs and a hot spring footbath. Tsubetsu Town offers a family bath and an outdoor bath to its guests.

Direct contact with trees

Coming into direct contact with trees allows participants to feel the warmth of the trunks and enjoy the textures of the different barks. During laboratory experiments (see pages 172–3), we found that contact with wood relaxes the brain and the body, so we hope in the future to clarify the relaxation effects that occur when coming into contact with trees during *shinrin-yoku*.

In Japan, cedar is a symbolic tree and many examples, like the huge cedar at the forest therapy base in Koya Town, are more than 500 years old. Natural beech forests in Japan, like the one at the base in Iiyama City, allow participants to soak up the mystical atmosphere these forests offer.

Stargazing

Due to the rapid increase of air pollution in urban areas in Japan, opportunities to observe the stars have been drastically reduced, so stargazing tours have become an attractive part of forest therapy programmes. The base at Achi Village was recognized by the Ministry of the Environment in 2006 as the best place in Japan to view the stars. Stargazing tours are also held in Okutama Town in the far west of Tokyo and Tsubetsu Town in the north of Hokkaido, with many people gathering to see the fantastic sights.

Sea of clouds

This phenomenon occurs at the Tsubetsu Town base and is a good example of a forest therapy base using its own unique natural resources to offer participants unusual activities. Participants are taken to the high-altitude Tsubetsu Pass to view the clouds below, which create the impression of a sea. Viewing the sea of clouds together with the sunrise is a majestic sight. Participants drink tea while enjoying the view as the sun rises.

Snow-covered mountains

Many forest therapy walking courses close when snow falls, but some bases are starting to develop snow-covered mountain forest therapy programmes. Our park therapy experiments showed that even when the outside temperature is low, if subjects are wearing warm clothing, parasympathetic nerve activity (known to increase during relaxation) still increases during walking in the park.[41] Therefore we can expect that the relaxation effect will be the same during snow-covered mountain forest therapy.

Nordic walking

The base at Tome City is now developing a Nordic walking activity for elderly people, using ski poles for support. Japan's population continues to age and ensuring a good quality of life for elderly people is a pressing issue. Activities such as this can help with relaxation and wellbeing.

Cherry blossom viewing

Cherry blossom, which heralds the coming of spring, is an extremely significant flower in Japan. Blossom viewing is a highly regarded activity that is celebrated all over the country. Blossom plays an important role in Japanese culture and features in many famous poems and other works of art.

The cherry tree at Motosu City, which is known as *Usuzumi Zakura*, is thought to be 1,500 years old. With a height of 16.3m (53ft) and a trunk diameter of 9.9m (32ft), it is classified as one of the three great cherry trees of Japan. Many people come to view this tree in blossom, as part of a forest therapy programme.

Flowers and forests

The combination of a serene forest and bright flowers such as azaleas as an under-storey, is an important element of many forest therapy programmes. Akagi Nature Park and Koya Town are celebrated for their displays of wonderful seasonal flowers, which make forest therapy at these bases an even more memorable and enjoyable experience.

Terraced rice fields

Terraced rice fields are an evocative part of the Japanese countryside, enhancing the already beautiful mountain landscapes, so they make attractive additions to forest therapy programmes. The base at Ukiha City integrates rice fields into its forest therapy activities.

Tea picking

Green tea is an integral part of everyday life for Japanese people and has great cultural significance in tea ceremonies. In the tea growing area of Yamakita Town, a unique tea picking course has been developed as part of the forest therapy programme there, allowing participants to enjoy stimulation of all five senses while picking tea.

Music concerts

The aural and visual stimulation of watching live musicians play music in a beautiful forest setting has the potential to increase the therapeutic effects of forest therapy. The forest therapy centres at Heavens Sonohara, Tsubetsu Town and Kirishima City offer concerts as part of their forest therapy programmes.

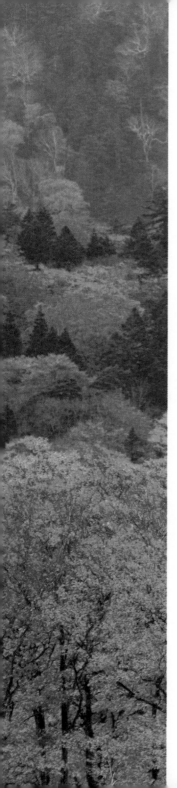

Autumn foliage

Colourful autumn foliage is another seasonal event, like cherry blossom viewing, which allows forest therapy participants to experience the seasons through nature. Akagi Nature Park and Jinsekikogen Town are widely celebrated for their autumn foliage, which attracts visitors from far and wide.

Aroma workshops

Olfactory stimuli (aromas) strongly affect the limbic system, which governs emotions, making aroma workshops an effective part of forest therapy programmes. These activities are particularly popular among women and include aroma creation and essential oil extraction. The centres at Heavens Sonohara and Tsubetsu Town offer popular courses.

Horse riding and dog therapy

The forest therapy bases at Jinsekikogen Town and Ueno Village are developing a unique venture to increase the effects of forest therapy through contact with animals such as dogs and horses. Research has shown that coming into contact with animals can have a relaxing effect on people so these are worthwhile activities.

Programmes for children

Some forest therapy centres, such as those in Tsu City and Tsubetsu Town, offer programmes designed especially for children, and include activities such as making water shoots, catching fish and tree climbing.

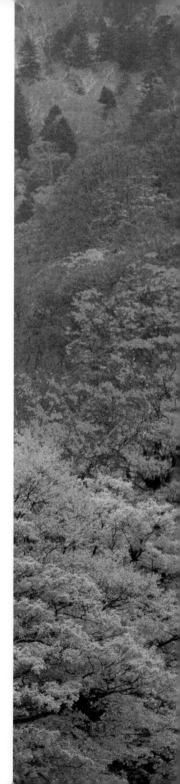

What is the best nature therapy for you?

There is a wide variety of nature therapies available, from residential forest therapy programmes, half-day and day-long walks, park therapy, indoor essential oil therapy, forest scenery programmes, forest sounds and a whole range of other activities described on the previous pages. This may sound a little vague, but you should choose the nature therapy that appeals to you most. Research has shown that there is a correlation between the activities you enjoy and the physiological relaxation effects they provide. In other words, the more you are enjoying an activity, the greater its benefits will be.

We conducted experiments where subjects listened to the sound of a murmuring forest stream through speakers while we measured their brain activity and blood pressure. We asked them to rate their enjoyment of the sound and they reported a variety of reactions, from an impression of comfort to not feeling anything in particular. There was no physiological relaxation effect in the subjects who did not feel anything in particular, but in the subjects who felt comfort from the sound, we found a calming of prefrontal brain activity, a reduction in blood pressure and a physiological relaxation effect.

We found the same result with visual stimulation, when subjects are asked to look at something rather than listen to a sound, and even with the smell of freshly ground coffee beans. If subjects enjoyed the experience, it had a calming effect; if they didn't feel anything special, it had no effect. Many of our experiments into natural stimuli have demonstrated this relationship between a feeling of comfort/enjoyment and physiological relaxation effects. If a person is taking part in a nature therapy feeling comfortable and relaxed, their body is also experiencing relaxation.

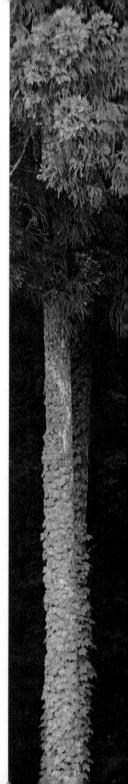

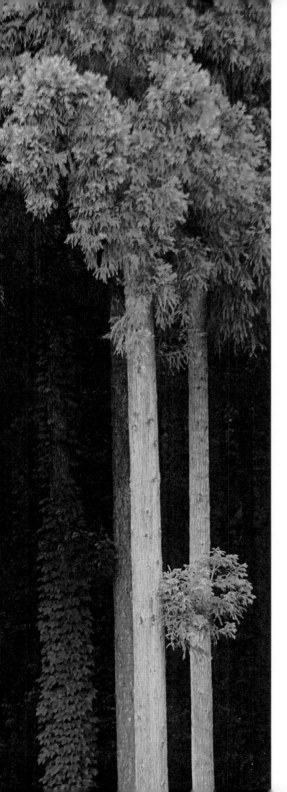

When choosing a therapy to try,
I recommend that you do some
research on the internet and get an
intuitive feel for what might work for
you. For example, for those who are
interested in aromas, a therapy using
essential oils will be effective. Our
experiments showed that the aroma
from the wood and leaves of pine
trees and Japanese cypresses calmed
brain activity and boosted the
parasympathetic nerve activity that
increases during relaxation.

Those people who gain pleasure
from gardening or bonsai could
concentrate on therapies based around
these activities, while others might be
attracted to full immersion in a forest.
The advice is, if you like the idea of it,
it is likely to work for you.

So please make use of the nature that
appeals to you, to help you enjoy a
full and happy life.

Forest therapy bases in Japan

As we have seen, Japan is a densely forested, mountainous country with many different climatic zones and many different types of forest. Currently, there are 63 forest therapy bases in Japan, from Hokkaido to Okinawa. The four forest therapy bases I have chosen here as examples have all been shown to have beneficial physiological relaxation effects by research conducted there.

AKASAWA NATURAL RECREATIONAL FOREST

This base, in Agematsu Town in Nagano Prefecture, is the birthplace of *shinrin-yoku* and is situated in a natural forest of Japanese cypresses, many over 300 years old. Certified forest therapy sessions have been held here since 2005 and this is one of the country's leading forest therapy bases.

The base offers a two-day health check and forest therapy programme, which includes a physical examination at the start, a guided walk in the forest with a doctor and a thorough health check. One of the most popular features of the base is a forest railway which runs alongside the walking trail. In the summer, there are water activities in the river that runs through the forest.

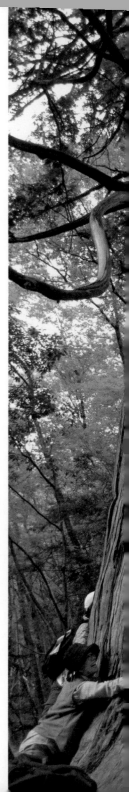

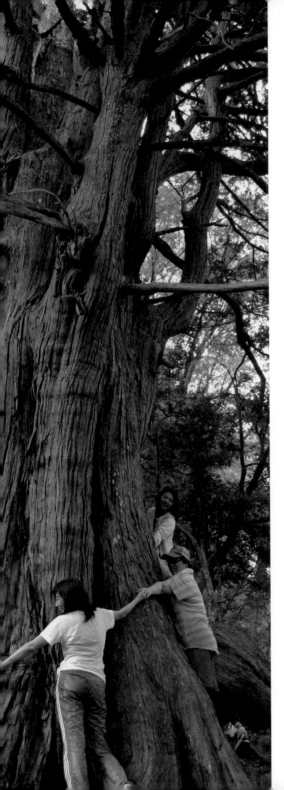

OKUTAMA TOWN, TOKYO

Okutama Town is on the western edge of Tokyo and is abundant in nature. It is renowned for having the largest number of huge trees in Japan and was recognized as a forest therapy base in 2008. The activities developed here form the model for forest therapy bases nationwide.

In addition to typical forest therapy sessions, the base offers a wide range of activities, including stargazing, meditation, yoga, soba-noodle making and pottery workshops. The following is an example of a forest therapy programme.

DAY ONE

10.30 Forest therapy (walking and contact with huge trees) and refreshments
12.30 Soba-noodle making
13.45 Pottery workshop
19.30 Stargazing

DAY TWO

09.50 Forest therapy (meditation)
10.50 Forest therapy (yoga)
12.30 Forest therapy and refreshments

CHIZU TOWN

Chizu Town in Tottori Prefecture is well known as a forest town because more than 90 per cent of its total area is forested. The town became a forest therapy base in 2010 with the aim of promoting forest therapy and revitalizing the region using a fusion of science and forest therapy. I have conducted some of my research here.

The base offers very good one-day programmes, but there is a particular focus on two-day and three-day corporate training programmes, using forest therapy to aid relaxation and wellbeing.

NONNO NO MORI NATURE CENTRE

Located in Tsubetsu Town on the island of Hokkaido, this base offers a variety of programmes that focus on the changing of the seasons, making full use of Hokkaido's rich natural environment. Much of the therapy is designed to stimulate the five senses, and includes snow shoe sessions in winter, lying in hammocks in the snow, stargazing at night, firefly observation, children's tree-climbing sessions and a sea-of-clouds tour which takes participants up over the Tsubetsu Pass to view the clouds below. There are also plans to include extraction of forest fragrances using a still and forest concerts played by musicians. The following programme is held at Nonno No Mori in the summer months:

DAY ONE

16.00 Forest therapy
20.30 Firefly observation in the forest, or stargazing guided tour

DAY TWO

06.00 Tsubetsu Pass sea-of-clouds tour
10.30 Forest aromatherapy
13.30 Forest concert

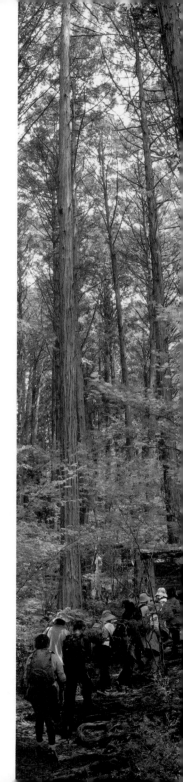

Walk mindfully

The practice of *shinrin-yoku* is based on walking through the forest at a gentle pace for two hours or more. Keeping your phone switched off allows time to soak up the environment around you and come into the here and now. The phrase *shikan shouyou* means "nothing but wandering along", something we rarely get a chance to do, but which is very beneficial.

Feel your feet touching the ground. The movement of your muscles. The constant balancing and rebalancing of the body. Pay attention to any areas of stiffness or pain in the body and consciously relax them.

Become aware of your present mental and emotional states. Notice your state of mind. Is it calm or busy, cloudy or focused? Where is your mind?

Be aware of your location in space, the sounds around you and the air temperature.

Pay attention to the experience of walking and keep your awareness engaged in this experience.

Be aware of the beginning, the middle and the end of your stepping.

Walk as silently as possible.

Allow your awareness to move up through every part of your body, noticing the sensations as you walk. Gradually scan all parts of your body as you bring your attention to the ankles, skin, calves, knees, thighs, hips, pelvis, back, chest, shoulders, arms, neck and head.

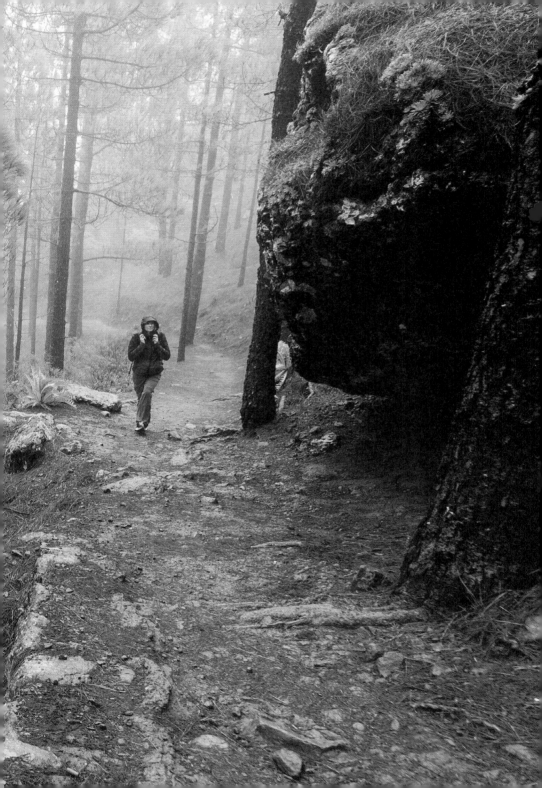

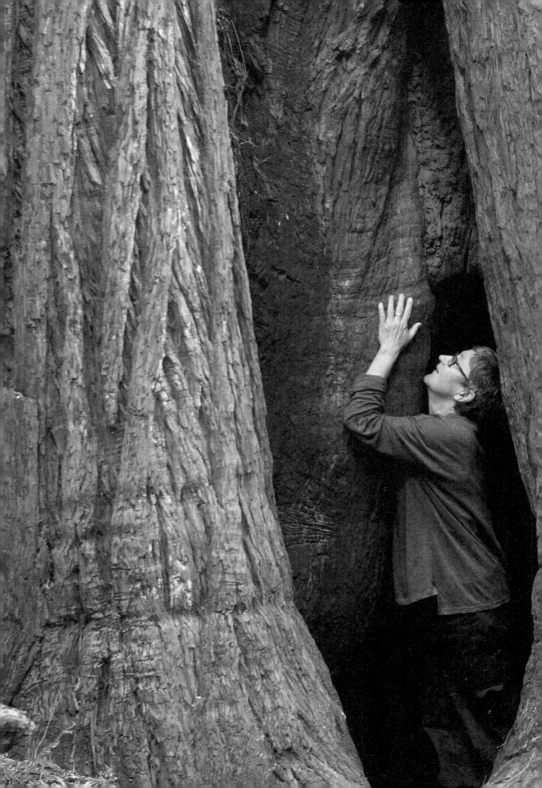

Use the five senses

Switch off your phone and let nature calm your body and mind through all five senses.

See all the colours and shapes and movement in the trees. Look closely at the details of the leaves and bark. Look up through the canopy to the sky.

Take in all the aromas of nature around you, the earth waking up in spring or leaves returning to the soil in autumn. The smell of a crisp winter's day, or a warm afternoon in late summer laden with the smell of ripening berries.

Listen to the sounds of nature, the birds, the breeze through the trees, the rustle of leaves underfoot.

Touch the trees with all their textures, feel the cool water of a stream. Hugging a tree will give you an immediate sense of connection to nature.

Food eaten outdoors really does taste better, so take a picnic and a flask of tea. Enjoy the opportunity to sit and just be with nature for a while.

Meditate

Meditating in nature is another way to amplify the positive effects of the environment around you.

Meditation and mindfulness are excellent for calming the mind by bringing awareness and attention into the present moment. You don't need to empty your mind to enjoy the benefits of meditation; it is simply a case of observing the mind and bringing it back into awareness when you find it wandering off.

A simple meditation

1 Find a comfortable place to sit.

2 Either close your eyes or lower them to rest gently on a spot about a metre in front of you on the ground.

3 Spend a few minutes bringing your full attention to your breath, breathing naturally in and out through your nose. Just notice the breath – in and out.

4 Now bring your attention to the soles of your feet and just imagine them fully relaxed. Gradually bring your relaxed attention through your feet up into your ankles and calves. Take time to simply check in with every part of your body, breathing a feeling of relaxation into every muscle and place of tension.

5 When you reach the very top of your head, just bring your attention fully back to the breath, gently in and gently out. Imagine inhaling nature, then as you breathe out let go of any remaining tension.

6 Remain meditating on the breath for as long as you wish. When you are ready, take a count of five to bring your attention back to your surroundings. If your eyes were closed, gently open them.

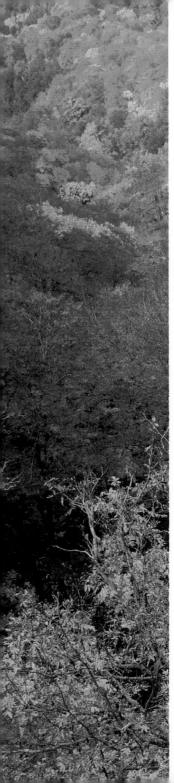

Stretch

Many of us live a more sedentary life than our bodies were designed for. Stretching is an excellent, gentle way to get the body moving. Being in nature is a body–mind activity, and by stretching mindfully you bring your awareness back into your body rather than concentrating on the thoughts in your mind, thereby encouraging your body back to its natural state.

Chest opener

Clasp your hands together behind your head. Inhale and feel your chest rise, pulling your elbows back and pressing your head into your hands. Exhale and release, then repeat as often as you like, using smooth, controlled movements and breathing slowly and deeply.

Standing hip stretch

Cross your left ankle over your right thigh and, if you can, bend your right leg to increase the stretch in your hip and bottom. Extend your arms in front of you to help you balance, or use a nearby tree for support. Fix your gaze on a spot in front of you and breathe smoothly and deeply. Hold the position for 30–60 seconds, then repeat on the other side.

Quad stretch

Grasp your right foot or ankle with your right hand and gently pull your heel toward your bottom. Press to increase the stretch in your right hip, trying to keep your knees together. Hold for 30–60 seconds, then repeat on the other side.

Hamstring stretch

Extend your right leg out in front of you with your foot flexed, balancing on your left leg. Keeping your back straight and chest lifted, slowly lean forwards, hinging at the hips, to increase the stretch. Breathe deeply for 30–60 seconds, then release and repeat on the other side.

Side bend

Stand with your feet hip-width apart and place your palms together over your head. Inhale and reach up to elongate your spine. As you exhale, reach over to your right, keeping your chest open and allowing your hips move to the left a little. As you inhale, release the stretch, then deepen the stretch again as you exhale. Repeat four or five times, slowly moving with your breath. Repeat the exercise on the other side.

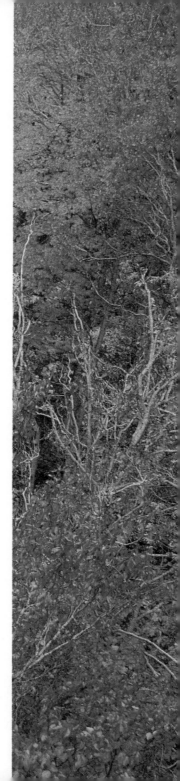

Stargaze

If you are able to walk safely in a forest at night, a whole host of different experiences will greet your senses, and stargazing is one of the most remarkable.

As it waxes and wanes through the month, the moon reminds us of the rhythms of nature, while the stars give us a sense of perspective.

According to researchers from the University of California, Irvine, feeling a sense of awe takes our minds off our personal problems and promotes an increase in cooperation and connection with others.

Lie down on a mat or in a hammock and scan the sky for shooting stars. If it is a cold night, take a cosy blanket to keep you feeling comfortable and relaxed.

Breathe

Absorb the atmosphere of the forest while gazing at the stars, with these simple breathing exercises.

EQUAL BREATHING Breathe in through your nose for a count of 4, then out through your nose for a count of 4. Breathe in this way for 5 minutes. If you can increase the count, then do so.

ABDOMINAL BREATHING Place one hand on your abdomen and one hand on your chest. Breathe in through your nose into your abdomen until you feel your lungs expand, then gently breathe out through your nose. Continue the exercise for up to 10 minutes.

"Allow nature's peace to flow into you
as sunshine flows into trees"

— JOHN MUIR

Spend time in a hammock

Resting while immersed in nature is extremely relaxing and restorative.

The power of quality rest is often underestimated and undervalued, but now scientists are discovering that good sleep and rest is very important to health and a sense of wellbeing.

If you don't have a hammock, lay a mat or folded blanket on the ground. Alternatively, use a reclining sun lounger. If the weather is cold, dress up warm and take a blanket to snuggle under.

Spending time in nature increases activity in the parasympathetic nervous system, helping the body to "rest and digest". Encouraging the body to regulate itself naturally in this way helps to promote and maintain good health.

Poor sleep is linked to physical problems such as a weakened immunity, and mental health problems such as anxiety and depression. Feeling rested contributes to our sense of feeling well and also builds up our resources for dealing with the challenges of life.

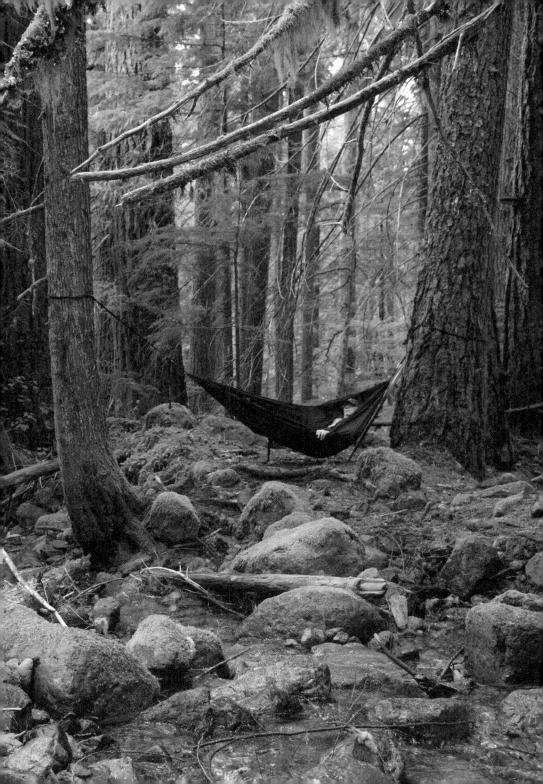

Learn

Nature is an excellent place for play and education. From the physical agility and resilience developed by climbing trees, to the innovation of building camps, to learning the names of trees, birds and butterflies, the forest offers children so many ways to grow.

> "Look deep into nature, and then you will understand everything better"
>
> — ALBERT EINSTEIN

Children who spend regular time in nature on average experience an increase in self-confidence, problem-solving skills, motor skills and the capacity to learn.

Developing an early appreciation of nature sets up a positive relationship for life, so that nature will continue to be a source of relaxation and connection throughout adulthood.

Even children are feeling the effects of today's modern world, with rates of depression and stress among young people increasing rapidly. Increased pressure to study and the rise in use of technology such as smartphones is leaving our children feeling frazzled. Time in nature is just as valuable to children as it is to adults.

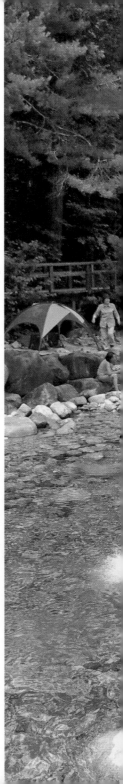

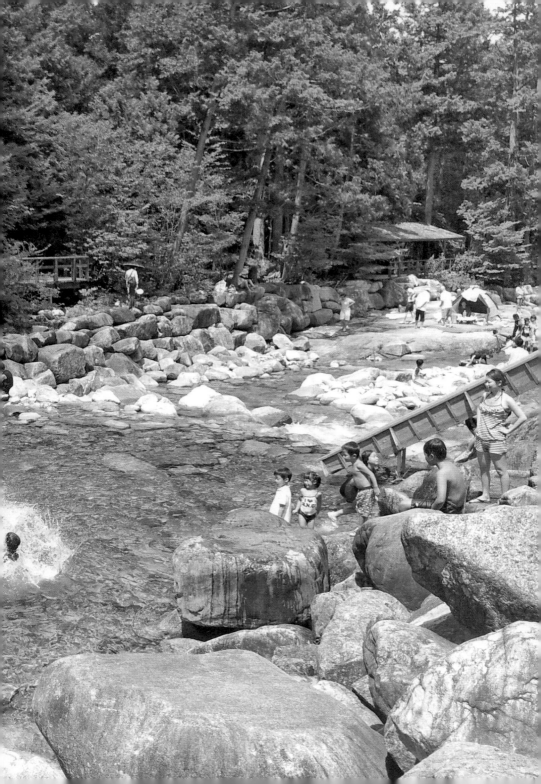

"Art takes nature
as its model"

— ARISTOTLE

Create

Creativity is a receptive process and being in nature encourages receptivity. Many writers over the ages have described walking through the woods, and nature itself has inspired so many poems and beautiful pieces of prose.

Take a sketchbook and pencil and find a comfortable place to sit. Draw what you see, whether an overall scene of the forest or a detail of a leaf. Don't feel self-conscious; you don't have to show it to anybody else.

Nature is a wonderful place for journal writing and exploring how you are feeling. When you are in a relaxed state you can consider things with more perspective and open up to new ideas.

The art of wood carving is growing in popularity again. Working with the materials of nature helps us to nurture a relationship with nature. The same is true for pottery; using your hands to create rather than type is refreshing both physically and mentally.

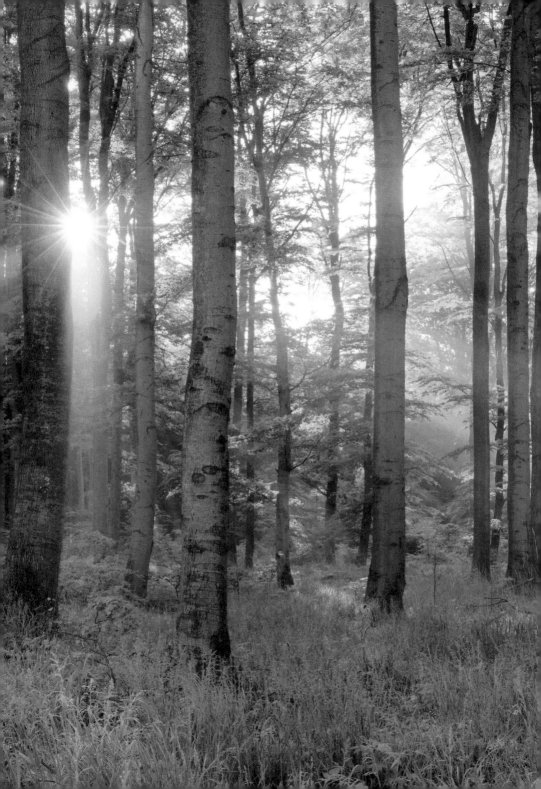

KOMOREBI 木漏れ日

"The interplay
of the light and
the leaves when
sunlight filters
through the trees"

CHAPTER 4

Bringing the Forest Closer to Home

森林をもっと身近に

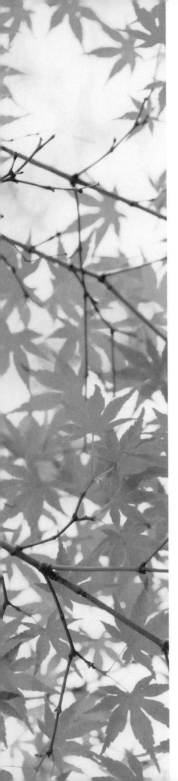

Not all of us have access to a natural forest where we can harness the benefits of *shinrin-yoku* on a regular basis, so how can we use the knowledge we now have about the wonderfully relaxing effects of nature to improve our health and wellbeing wherever we are?

Most cities and urban areas do have pockets of nature, whether it's the local park, an area of waste ground or an overgrown path down the side of a canal. Any space where there are plants growing can offer relaxation effects to those who are prepared to seek them out and spend time there. Interest in urban nature is on the increase, so you might well find clubs that organize walks or nature-watching trips to make the most of the green spaces on offer.

However, finding green spaces isn't always the problem; many of us are simply too busy to put aside time for ourselves, giving our minds and bodies no chance to unwind. So how can we bring the stress-relieving benefits of nature closer to the places we spend most of our time – our homes and workplaces?

As we will see in chapter 5, many elements of nature have the same beneficial effects as *shinrin-yoku*, including wooden objects and decor, ornamental plants in the house or garden, a vase of fresh flowers and even the aroma of essential oils derived from plants. This chapter offers ideas on how you can bring the forest closer to home and enjoy the relaxing benefits of nature every day.

Urban nature

Currently, just over half of the world's population lives in urban areas and this is expected to reach two-thirds by 2050.

Nature has an important part to play in helping to make cities sustainable and healthy places in which to live and work. In Singapore, for example, wooded areas make up almost 30 per cent of the city and there are plans to expand the green spaces so that, by 2030, 85 per cent of residents live within 400m (437 yards) of a park. Other green cities around the world – with over 20 per cent green space – include Vancouver, Sacramento, Frankfurt, Geneva, Amsterdam and Seattle.

City planners all over the globe are becoming aware of the importance of nature. There are many exciting projects where nature has helped to transform once-derelict city spaces, such as the High Line in New York City, which has become one of the most popular destinations in the city, and the Seoullo garden walkway in Seoul which brought 24,000 plants to a disused highway. In Munich's English Garden, there is a short man-made river called the Eisbach (German for "ice brook") in which city dwellers can go swimming.

Similarly, the swimming ponds on Hampstead Heath in London have provided an oasis of nature and wild swimming for Londoners since the early 18th century. Even in cities that are apparently "full", there are innovative plans to create nature corridors, such as a network of rooftop and ground-level gardens in the centre of Barcelona.

You only need to glance at a city park on a warm day to see how much people appreciate these green spaces as places to sit and eat their lunch, take a break or go for some exercise. As the experiments in chapter 5 suggest, walking through a city park has a calming effect on the mind and body. It makes common sense, but now the scientific evidence is helping to make the case for the importance of including nature in urban planning, for both the mental and physical health of the residents.

New York's High Line has transformed an abandoned railroad spur on the west side of Manhattan, making it one of the most popular destinations in the city.

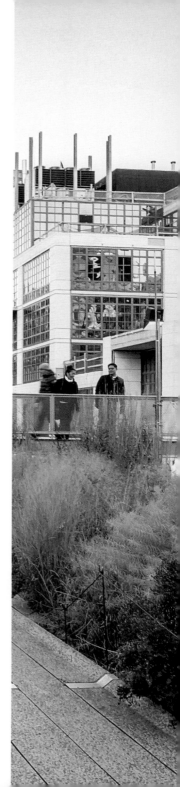

NATURE AND ARCHITECTURE

As well as urban parks, there are exciting examples of architecture and design that integrate city living with nature. "Living walls" allow for the inclusion of a large number of plants in very little space, providing a stunning aesthetic to a building as well as benefitting both humans and the environment. And rooftop gardens are increasingly providing the opportunity to create green spaces in urban settings. Offices can often be rather sterile unnatural environments and so it can make a significant difference to be able to access nature easily on the roof.

Likewise, architects designing new schools are increasingly looking at ways to connect education with nature, creating green corridors between buildings and kitchen gardens for the children to be involved with growing vegetables and learning about food.

COMMUNITY GARDENING AND CITY FARMS

All over the world there are community gardening projects in towns and cities, usually focused on growing fruit and vegetables. These projects help to bring communities together and introduce nature into people's everyday lives.

Brooklyn Grange has 1 hectare (2.5 acres) of rooftop soil farms in New York City, growing 22,650kg (50,000lb) of fresh produce each year for local farmers' markets and restaurants, and provides immersive workshops for thousands of school students. And networks of urban beekeepers are growing in numbers across many towns and cities, with gardeners being encouraged to grow bee-friendly plants and flowers.

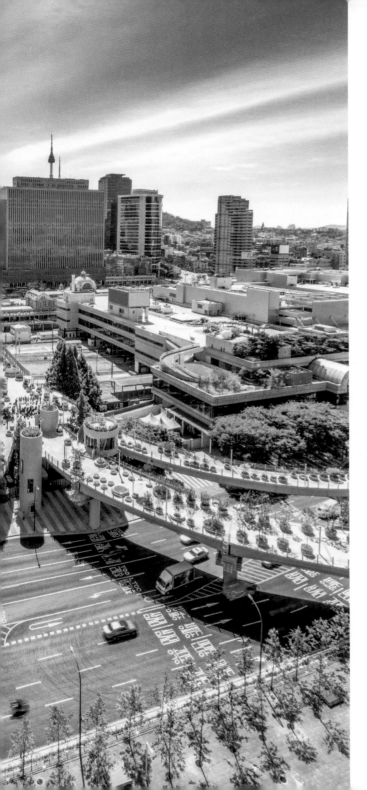

Seoullo Skygarden is a new pedestrian walkway built on what was a dangerous old overpass in Seoul, South Korea's capital city.

Wood therapy

Research has shown that if we find them pleasing, wooden elements used in the home and workplace – in the form of furniture, fixings and features – can offer relaxation benefits when we look at the wood, touch it or smell it.

Wood can be introduced into the home in many ways and has always been popular as an architectural element in the form of wooden panels, beams, kitchen worktops and floors. In our research, we found that the amount of wood used in a room can affect its relaxation benefits, and these benefits are linked to how much the subjects liked or felt comfortable in the room. So the message is, if you like it, it is probably benefitting you.

TREATED VS UNTREATED WOOD

We found that the relaxing benefits of tactile stimulation – simply touching wood – are affected by any coating on the wood, such as varnish. We asked blindfolded subjects to lay their palms on squares of white oak wood, rather like offcuts of a kitchen worktop, for 90 seconds. If the wood was untreated, the subjects experienced reduced brain activity, increased parasympathetic nervous activity, reduced sympathetic nervous activity and lower heart rate, all signs of relaxation. These effects were much reduced if the wood had been treated with a urethane- or vitreous-based coating.[49]

THE AROMA OF WOOD

We will see in chapter 5 that inhaling the aroma of naturally dried wood calms prefrontal brain activity and relaxes the human body (see pages 172–3). We can interpret this as a return to a natural state of being through the calming of a brain that is habitually overworked by our artificial environment. The same effect has been shown when people inhale the aroma of essential oils derived from trees, but the effect is most pronounced when the person likes the aroma. See page 116 for more information about how to use essential oils.

INTRODUCING WOOD INTO YOUR LIFE

Wood is a useful material which can be used to make many different elements in the home or workplace. Don't forget to choose things you like; the relaxation effects only work if you like the wood.

- Natural wood floors can look contemporary as well as rustic.

- Wood panelling softens the look of a room, but remember to leave it unpainted.

- Wooden worktops and cabinets can make a kitchen feel warmer. Even when wooden surfaces are treated to protect them against moisture, thereby reducing the effects of touching them, you will still benefit from looking at them.

- Choose wood that has been dried naturally, rather than heat-treated, to benefit from its aroma.

- Wooden furniture fits with many styles of decoration and offers an easy way to increase the amount of wood in a home or workplace.

- Leave beams exposed and untreated where possible.

- Choose wooden chopping boards, spoons, bowls and other utensils for the kitchen.

- Decorate your home with small wooden carvings and other decorative items.

- Use essential oils derived from trees to scent your home, bath or moisturizer.

JAPANESE CYPRESS BATHS

A popular way for Japanese people to enjoy wood therapy on a regular basis is by taking a cypress bath. These bathtubs are made from solid cypress wood. When it comes into contact with hot water, the wood produces a strong aroma of cypress, providing physical and mental relaxation. As with any contact with wood, the reason cypress baths are so relaxing is down to three things:

· **The aroma of the wood** produces a calming of prefrontal brain activity, which we can interpret as relaxation.

· **Contact with the wood** produces a calming of prefrontal brain activity and a rise in parasympathetic nerve activity – another physiological relaxation effect.

· **The sight of the wood** – people who like Japanese cypress wood experience a decrease in blood pressure when they see it, so it's likely that the sight of a cypress bath is relaxing to the bather.

SAUNAS AND BATH BARRELS

The "sauna" is a Finnish bathing ritual which is thousands of years old. You sit in a wood-panelled room heated by hot stones and enjoy intense heat. In Finland, saunas are said to be "a poor man's pharmacy" and cedar wood, which contains α-pinene (a wood oil compound shown to have a positive effect on parasympathetic nerve activity; see pages 172–3), is often used in their construction.

In Switzerland bath barrels made of wood are a traditional way to enjoy a *thermalbad* ("thermal bath"), and one of the most striking examples is in Zurich, where fresh thermal waters bubble straight into the public spa which has been converted from a brewery.

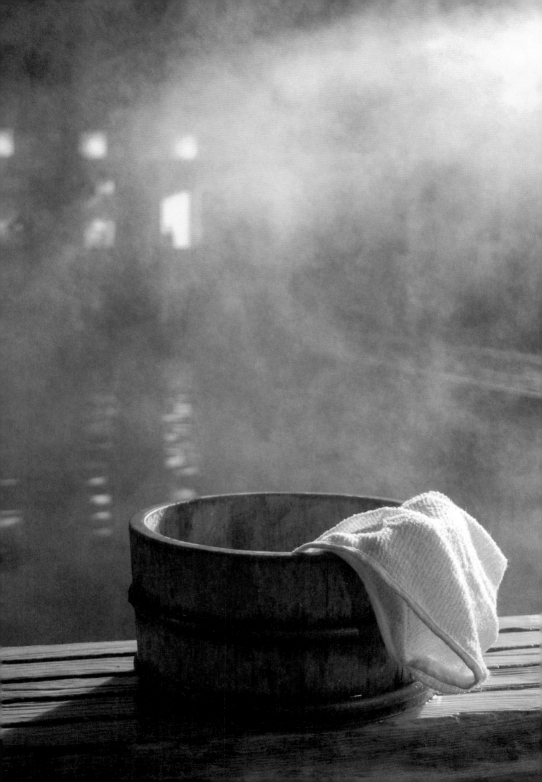

Bonsai

The art of growing miniature trees is most commonly associated with Japan, although the practice originated in China and spread through Korea to Japan around 1,000 years ago. The first dwarf trees occurred naturally, growing on rocky outcrops in the mountains of China, the harsh conditions and lack of soil stunting their growth.

Today, many different species are grown as bonsai, from cedar and juniper to maple and fig, some planted singly, others making up miniature landscapes with many trees potted together. Bonsai specimens can live for centuries, and they age in the same way as full-sized trees, becoming gnarly and more beautiful as they get older.

The traditional purposes of bonsai are contemplation for the viewer, and the gentle work and ingenuity required of the grower. As we will see in chapter 5, even simply sitting and looking at a bonsai tree (see pages 166–7) produces the same relaxation effects as walking in a forest, so bonsai can be an enjoyable and beneficial hobby and requires very little space. Tending a bonsai tree is a mindful activity that brings you into the present moment as you concentrate on the task in hand. Bringing nature into your daily life doesn't mean you need to go and find a forest; you can create your own forest at home on a miniature scale.

Like any form of gardening or flower arranging, bonsai allows us to connect with nature in a creative way. There is a sense of sculpting the tree while understanding its natural balance and the way it grows.

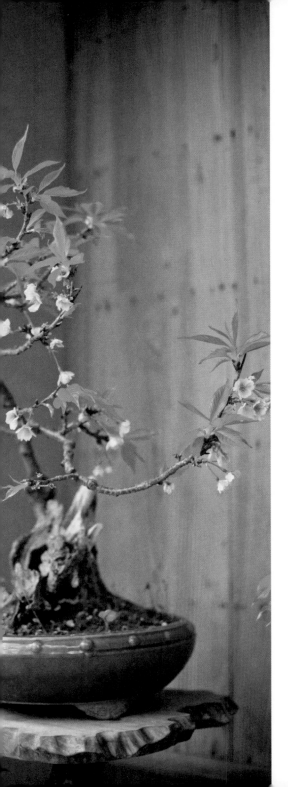

GROWING BONSAI

Bonsai specimens can be bought ready shaped, or you can raise them from scratch from a seed or sapling. Whichever route you take, your bonsai will need regular tending through pruning and shaping, a fascinating and pleasing process. Like most houseplants, it's a case of watering regularly, but not too much; feeding, but not too much; and lots of love and attention.

Plants and flowers

Most us intuitively understand that ornamental plants, whether outside or inside the home or workplace, do improve our sense of wellbeing and many studies have proved this. One of the experiments that is described in chapter 5 shows how when subjects simply sat and looked at a houseplant, they experienced both physiological and psychological relaxation (see pages 164–5). There are many ways to harness this effect, using plants both indoors and outdoors.

OUTDOOR SPACES

Those of us lucky enough to have a garden will recognize the restorative nature of its atmosphere, whether we are simply relaxing in it, or working to maintain it. Gardening therapy is becoming more and more popular, and some of the *shinrin-yoku* centres in Japan offer simple gardening tasks, such as repotting plants, as therapy to guests.

But even if you don't have a garden, you might be able to garden on a smaller scale by growing some plants in pots on a balcony, or perhaps fixing a window box outside to house a few ornamental plants or herbs. Spending time with plants really can improve your health and wellbeing.

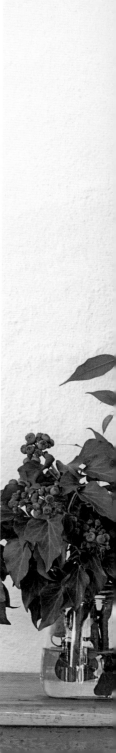

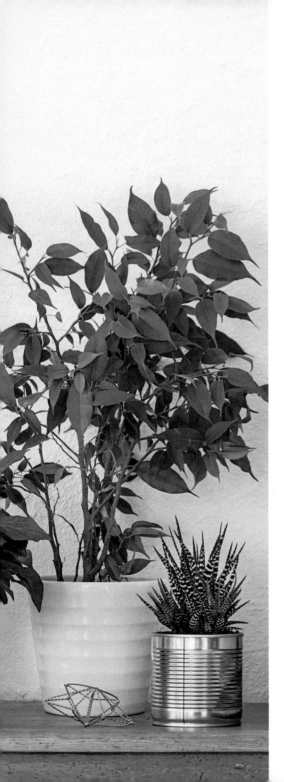

BRINGING NATURE INDOORS

Houseplants have been shown to relax the mind and body (see pages 164–5), so try to include them in as many rooms in your house as possible. There is a huge range of species on offer, from leafy foliage plants and colourful flowering plants to spiky cacti and smooth succulents.

When choosing plants for your home, pick something that will thrive there and continue to look attractive. Take into consideration the temperature, light levels, humidity and how much time you will have to care for your plants. It's unlikely that a sad and shrivelled houseplant will have the same relaxation effects as an attractive one.

How to fill your life with plants

When it comes to houseplants, the more the merrier, so be ingenious in finding places to keep them.

· A decorative plant on the kitchen table or dining table makes a nice centrepiece and gives you the opportunity to appreciate it up close.

· Group plants of different sizes together for greater impact. This allows you to include more plants in your home and creates a more cohesive design.

· Grow a selection of small plants in a terrarium if you are short of space. The even temperature and humidity offers beneficial growing conditions.

· If you don't have enough space on the floor or surfaces, create hanging displays by suspending small pots from hooks in the ceiling in macrame plant hangers.

· Climbing plants can save space too. Train them up a wall or a support pole in the pot.

· Many houseplants can be grown from seed, so this is a great way to fill your house with plants without spending too much money.

· Windowsills offer the bright conditions that many plants love, but be sure to choose sun-loving plants if your window faces south, and make sure plants are protected from draughts.

· Stand specimen plants on pedestals to increase their height and impact.

· Take a plant or two to work with you. Not only will it relax you, plants have also been shown to improve productivity.

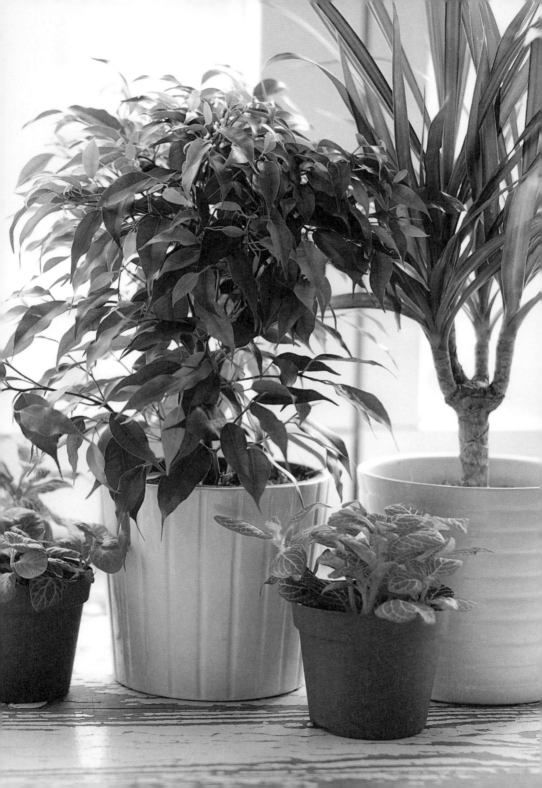

Cleaning the air

Houseplants don't just offer relaxation benefits in the home, it seems they also help to clean the air we breathe. Starting in the 1980s, a team of NASA scientists began a research programme, known as the Clean Air Study, to investigate ways to tackle "sick building syndrome". This phenomenon occurs when pollutants – from furniture, carpets and cleaning products – build up in a modern building without adequate ventilation, causing headaches, dizziness and nausea in its inhabitants.

The scientists found that potted houseplants can eliminate levels of benzene, formaldehyde and trichloroethylene from the air. The effect might in part be due to the micro-organisms in the potting compost, but different types of plant had different levels of effect. The following ten common houseplants have air-cleansing abilities:

- Areca palm (*Chrysalidocarpus lutescens*)
- Lady palm (*Rhapis excelsa*)
- Bamboo palm (*Chamaedorea seifrizii*)
- Rubber plant (*Ficus elastica*)
- Corn plant (*Dracaena fragrans*)
- English ivy (*Hedera helix*)
- Miniature date palm (*Phoenix roebelenii*)
- Long-leaved fig (*Ficus binnendijkii* 'Alii')
- Boston fern (*Nephrolepis exaltata* 'Bostoniensis')
- Peace lily (*Spathiphyllum wallisii*)

Fresh flower displays

As we will see in chapter 5, the sight of a simple bunch of fresh flowers relaxes the body (see pages 168–9) in the same way houseplants do. It's not difficult to buy a cheap bunch of flowers in the supermarket each week and place them on the dining table, or on your desk at work, where you can enjoy looking at them regularly. We conducted our experiments using an arrangement of unscented pink roses[62–65], but it is likely that all fresh flowers have the same effect. It is also likely that the relaxation effects offered by the flowers will be related to how much pleasure you get from looking at them, so choose flowers you like.

We also found that the benefit is increased if you can also enjoy the aroma of the flowers, so go for scented flowers such as lilies if possible.

Cut flowers have the advantage over houseplants in some ways because you'd don't need green fingers and they require very little care. You can place a vase of flowers in a position where houseplants would not thrive, and as long as they have fresh water, ideally with a little flower food added, they will look great for several days. Simply throw them away and replace them as they fade.

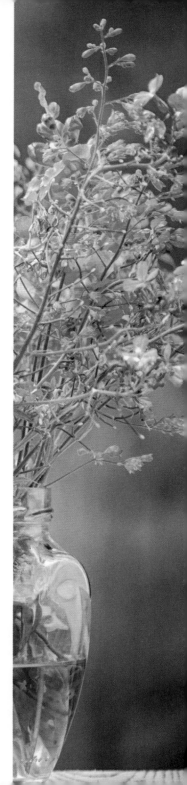

Essential oils

Essential oils are one of the easiest and most effective ways to bring the benefits of the forest into your home. If you have ever enjoyed the scent of a rose, you've experienced the aromatic qualities of essential oils. These natural aromatic compounds are found in the seeds, bark, stems, roots and flowers of plants. Essential oils give plants their distinctive aromas and have long been used in cooking, beauty treatments, as medicines and in relaxation therapies. Our experiments showed that essential flower oils, such as rose and orange, caused a physiological relaxation effect in subjects (see pages 170–1) and that many tree-derived oils have almost the same effect.

HOW TO USE ESSENTIAL OILS

· Place a few drops of your chosen oil in a simple diffusion device to scent your home.

· Mix a little oil with water in a spray bottle and mist over furniture, carpets or linens.

· Add some oil to a batch of laundry or to dryer sheets in your washer/dryer machine.

· Use in household surface cleaners.

· Add to massage oil. Dilute one drop of essential oil to three drops of a carrier oil like coconut oil to reduce the risk of skin sensitivity.

· Add a few drops of essential oil to a hot bath to enhance its relaxation effects.

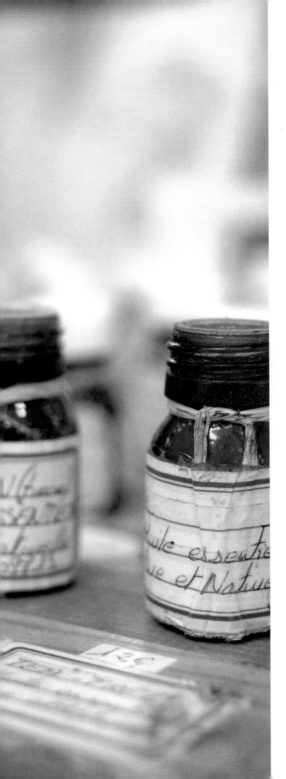

TREE-DERIVED ESSENTIAL OILS

We have done quite a bit of research on the physiological relaxation effects provided by tree-derived aromas, and results have shown that subjects experienced lower blood pressure, increases in parasympathetic nerve activity (known to increase during relaxation) and a calming of prefrontal brain activity when inhaling the aromas of all of the different types of wood we tested, which included Japanese cypress wood (hinoki),[52] Japanese cypress leaves,[53] Taiwanese hinoki wood[45] and thujopsis wood. This effect only worked, however, when the subject liked the aroma they were smelling; we found no effect among those that disliked it.

Since all of the woods we have investigated so far have resulted in these beneficial effects, choose any wood-derived essential oil you like, as long as you enjoy the aroma.

CEDARWOOD

The use of cedarwood oil, or cedar oil, dates back centuries. Its warm, woody scent is believed by many to soothe the mind and body, offering great relaxation benefits, and act as a grounding aroma which promotes feelings of vitality and wellness.

Plant description

Cedarwood oil comes from the red cedar (*Juniperus virginiana*), a coniferous evergreen tree native to eastern North America. It thrives at high altitude and grows up to 30m (100ft) tall.

Chemistry of cedarwood oil

Cedarwood oil contains a group of chemicals called sesquiterpenes. Essential oils that contain sesquiterpenes are empirically recognized for their ability to promote grounding and balance the emotions.

Uses and benefits

· Put three or four drops in a diffuser at the end of a long day to ground yourself and create a relaxing environment.

· To improve your exercise routine, massage one or two drops into your chest to boost vitality before a workout.

· When you find yourself distressed by unfamiliar situations, inhale the aroma to calm the mind.

· Diffuse cedarwood oil in your home, office or workspace to promote feelings of confidence and self-esteem.

DOUGLAS FIR

With its clean, fresh and woody aroma, Douglas fir oil is believed to promote a positive mood and improve focus and concentration. It is also used to cleanse and purify the skin and clear airways.

Plant description

Douglas fir (*Pseudotsuga menziesii*) is a coniferous tree which grows throughout North America. This tall, evergreen fir is often used as a Christmas tree. The sweet and refreshing oil smells of lemons.

Chemistry of Douglas fir oil

Douglas fir is rich in β-pinene, contributing to its ability to clear the airways. It also contains α-pinene, a compound we proved has relaxing benefits when inhaled on its own (see page 173).

Uses and benefits

· Combine with wild orange, lemon or bergamot oil in a diffuser to freshen the air, improve your mood and help you focus.

· Add a drop to your facial cleanser or body wash to cleanse your skin, relax and invigorate you at the same time.

· Rub two or three drops into your hands then inhale deeply if your nose is blocked.

· Combine one or two drops of Douglas fir oil with the same amount of wintergreen oil for a relaxing massage. Dilute with a little coconut oil to reduce the likelihood of skin sensitivity.

EUCALYPTUS

With its camphoraceous, minty aroma, eucalyptus is used to clear the mind and reduce tension. It is recommended for its purifying properties, which can be beneficial for the skin, and it is used to help clear the airways.

Plant description

Eucalyptus (*Eucalyptus radiata*) is a tall, evergreen tree growing up to 20m (50ft) in height and native to Australia.

Chemistry of eucalyptus oil

The main aroma compounds of eucalyptus oil are eucalyptol and α-terpineol, which open the airways, promoting easier breathing. They are also thought to induce relaxation, making eucalyptus an ideal massage oil.

Uses and benefits

· Combine a few drops with water in a spray bottle, adding the same quantity of lemon oil or peppermint oil too if you wish, and use it to wipe down kitchen or bathroom surfaces.

· Place a few drops in your hands while showering, hold over your nose and breathe deeply to invigorate and promote vitality.

· Use three or four drops in a diffuser to scent your room.

· Dilute one or two drops with some coconut oil and use for a relaxing massage.

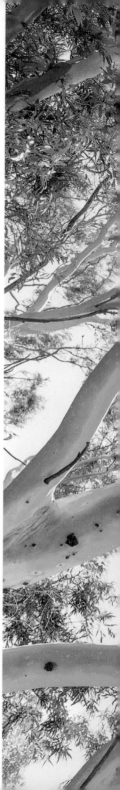

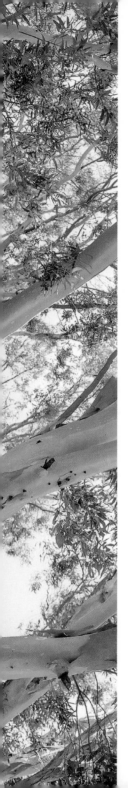

HIBA

With its strong, woody aroma that is similar to that of cedarwood oil, hiba oil has long been used for its antibacterial qualities and is an effective insect repellent. Our recent experiments, however, have shown that hiba can also be an effective tool to aid relaxation.

Plant description

Hiba (*Thujopsis dolabrata*) is a coniferous tree native to Japan, where it is known as *asunaro*. It is often found in gardens or planted close to temples.

Chemistry of hiba oil

The three major components in hiba oil are thujopsene, hinokitiol and β-dolabrin. Hinokitiol is known to have anti-fungal, antibacterial, anti-viral and anti-inflammatory effects.

Uses and benefits

· Use three or four drops in a hot bath to improve your mood after a hard day at work.

· Diffuse in your home, office or car as a deodorizer to keep nasty smells at bay and reduce feelings of stress and anxiety.

· Dilute a few drops in a base oil such as coconut and apply to the skin to reduce inflammation if you have eczema or psoriasis.

· Add a few drops to a spray bottle filled with water and use to keep insects away or to cleanse your home of bacteria.

SIBERIAN FIR

With its refreshing, piney and slightly balsamic scent, Siberian fir helps balance the emotions and soothes anxious feelings. It is empirically known for its calming and relaxing properties.

Plant description

Siberian fir (*Abies sibirica*) is a tall, evergreen conifer native to Russia and Canada. It is very hardy, surviving temperatures as low as −50°C (−58°F).

Chemistry of Siberian fir oil

Siberian fir contains high levels of bornyl acetate, a compound empirically known to promote physiological relaxation.

Uses and benefits

· Add a few drops to a neutral massage oil to soothe the skin and relax the body. This will be particularly beneficial after strenuous activity.

· Use three or four drops in a diffuser to promote easy breathing, while calming the emotions and providing a grounding effect.

· Siberian fir can help reduce stress during difficult times at home or work. Rub a few drops into the palms of your hands and inhale deeply.

· Dilute one or two drops in a little coconut oil to help soothe minor skin irritations.

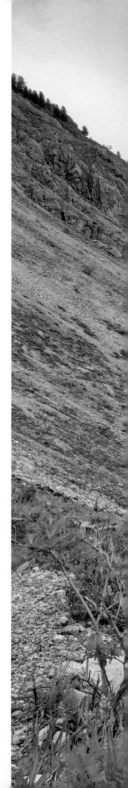

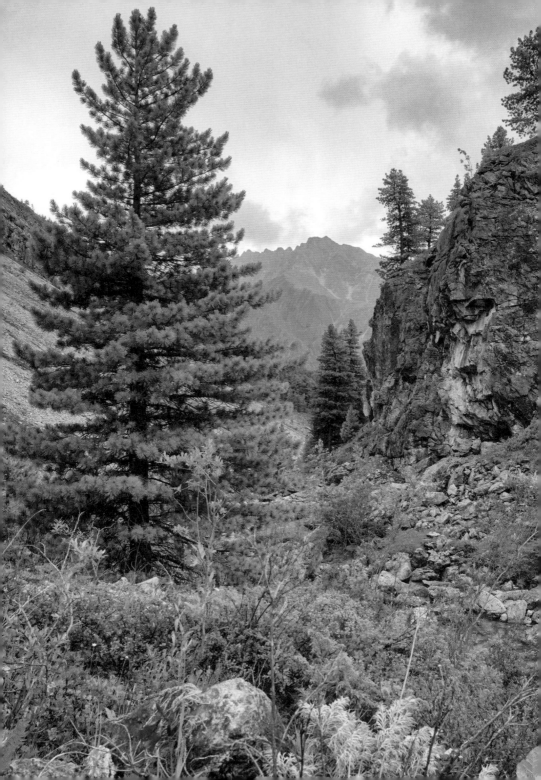

"The leaf of every tree
brings a message
from the unseen world.
Look, every falling leaf
is a blessing."

— RUMI

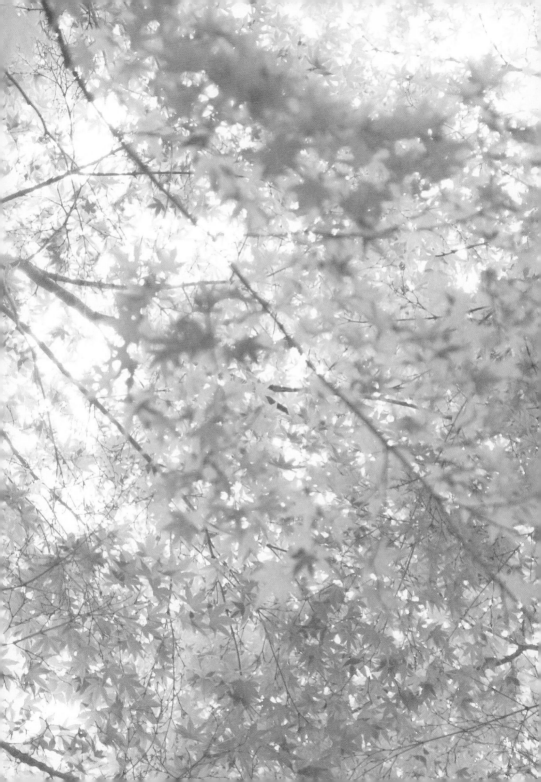

—

CHAPTER 5

The Science Behind Nature Therapy

自然セラピーの科学的背景

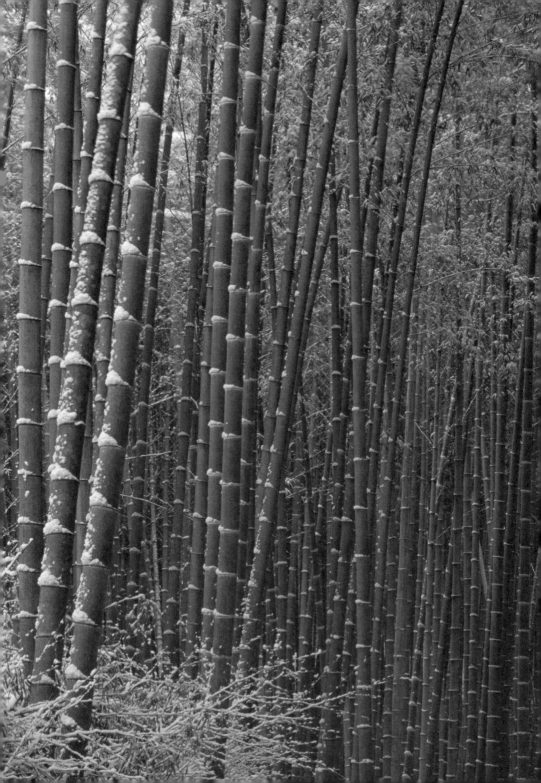

As we have evolved over millions of years, our bodies have become adapted to nature, so we automatically synchronize with the natural environment. When we are surrounded by nature, a feeling of comfort comes over us and our bodies become relaxed. Most of us would intuitively recognize this feeling, but until recently we haven't had any evidence to prove it. This is mainly because the right research techniques hadn't been established and, up until now, the only way to measure this relaxation effect was through questionnaires. Put simply, people were asked by researchers how relaxed they were feeling.

As we have already seen, scientists are now establishing more accurate ways to measure the physiological effects that nature therapies can have on our bodies, and new and revealing results are starting to emerge. This section explains how we can measure stress in the human body, then details some of my research into different nature therapies.

How can we measure stress?

In order to measure the relaxing effect of nature, we need to be able to measure accurately how stressed or relaxed our bodies are at any given time. There are four main ways that we can measure levels of stress and relaxation in the human body. They are:

· **By measuring brain activity** – as the level of relaxation increases, brain activity decreases

· **By measuring autonomic nervous activity** – as stress increases, activity in the sympathetic nervous system increases, while activity in the parasympathetic nervous system decreases

· **By measuring stress markers in saliva** – as stress increases, levels of these stress markers increase

· **By measuring immune activity** – as stress increases, the activity of natural killer (NK) cells decreases

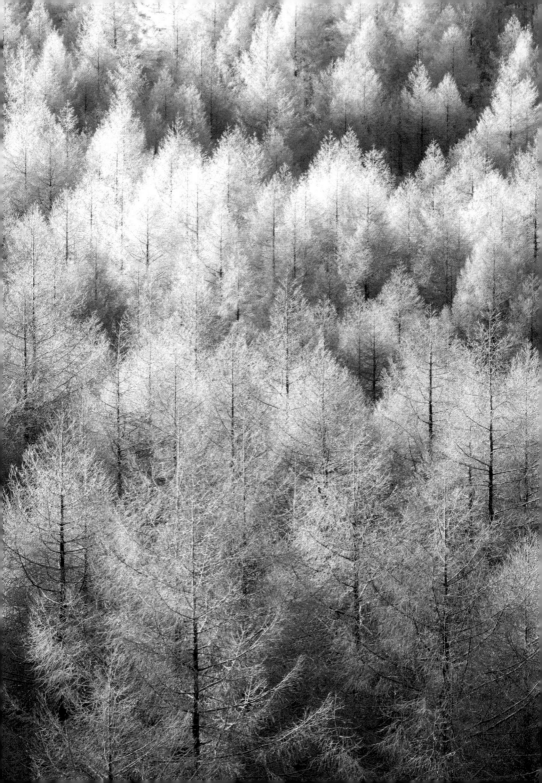

MEASURING BRAIN ACTIVITY

We know that activity in the prefrontal area of the brain decreases when we are in a state of relaxation. The brain needs oxygen to fuel this activity and the oxygen is carried to where it is needed by haemoglobin in the blood. We can therefore measure brain activity by measuring the concentration of oxygenated haemoglobin in the brain.

In nature therapy research, one of the best methods we have to measure the concentration of haemoglobin is near-infrared spectroscopy (NIRS). This is done by shining reddish, near-infrared light through the forehead into the brain. By measuring how much of the light is absorbed by the haemoglobin in the blood, we can measure the concentration of haemoglobin and therefore the level of activity in the brain.

Scientists have developed a small, lightweight and portable NIRS machine that allows measurements to be taken during therapy sessions in a forest. Although sensors have to be attached to the left and right of the subject's forehead, the process only takes about 20 seconds, causing minimal disruption.

Brain activity can also be measured using time-resolved spectroscopy (TRS). The major advantage of this method is that it can take absolute measurements of brain activity. Other methods, including near-infrared spectroscopy, can only measure increases or decreases in brain activity during a session when the sensors are in position. Once the sensors are removed, measurements cannot be compared to the next session so we cannot make comparisons of a subject's brain activity over a period of days or weeks. Time-resolved spectroscopy, however, does allow us to measure variation over long periods of time.

**Near-infrared light shining
on blood vessels**

**Near-infrared light
not absorbed**

Water

Blood low in
oxygenated haemoglobin

Blood rich in
oxygenated haemoglobin

This diagram shows the
principle of near-infrared
spectroscopy. Reddish
light is shone on the blood
vessels in the brain. The
amount of light absorbed
by the blood indicates
the concentration of
oxygenated haemoglobin,
and therefore the level
of activity in that part of
the brain.

MEASURING AUTONOMIC NERVOUS ACTIVITY

We know that activity in our parasympathetic nervous systems increases when we are relaxed, while that in our sympathetic nervous systems increases during periods of stress. We can therefore measure the activity in these systems to measure how stressed or relaxed we are, and we do this by measuring heart rate.

While we may think that our hearts beat regularly, in fact the period of time between beats varies. By analyzing this variability, we can now produce measurements of parasympathetic and sympathetic nervous activity. This method is called heart rate variability (HRV) and offers a sensitive record of relaxation and stress in the human body.

We usually measure HRV using a device that senses pulse waves in the blood vessels in the fingers. The intervals between these pulse waves are known to mirror the intervals between heartbeats. This is an easy way to record HRV as measurements are taken simply by placing a fingertip on the device.

In the past we could only measure autonomic nervous activity using the traditional methods of taking blood pressure and heart rate (pulse rate) measurements, but these methods can only show combined parasympathetic and sympathetic nervous activity. Heart rate variability is a much more useful method because it can measure the two things separately. In nature therapy research, we use all three different measurement methods to get a clearer picture: heart rate variability, blood pressure and heart rate (pulse rate).

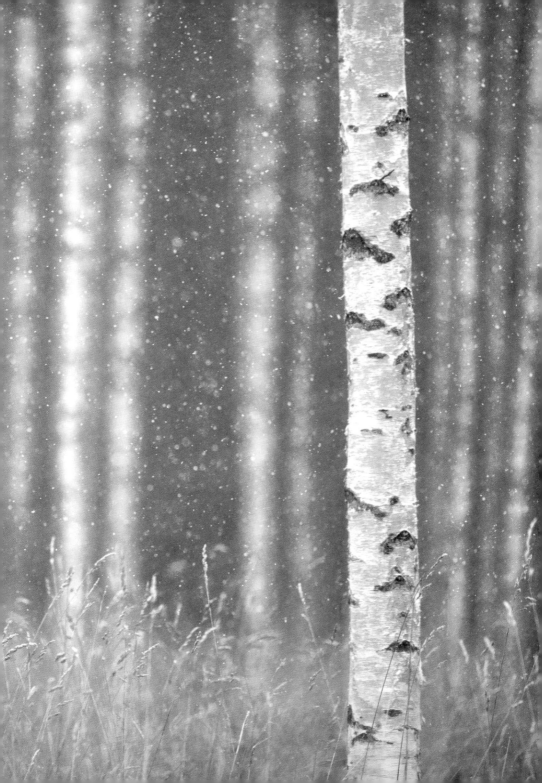

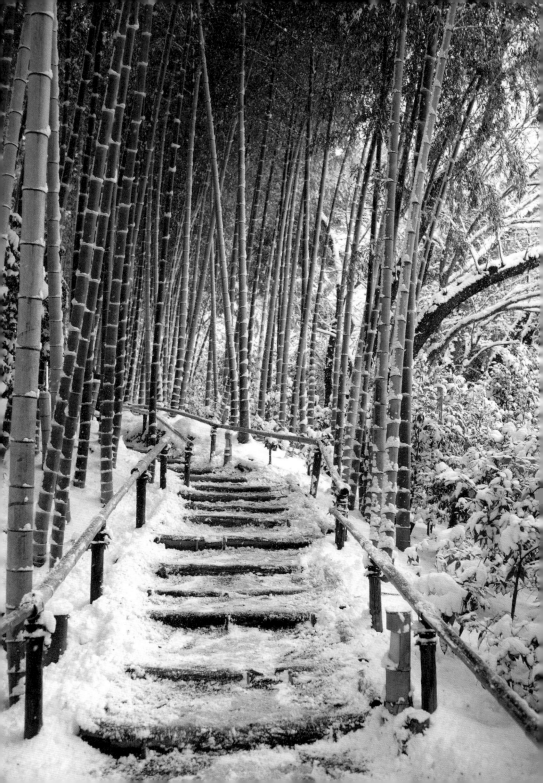

MEASURING STRESS MARKERS IN SALIVA

Cortisol is a hormone that is released by the adrenal gland in times of stress. Levels of cortisol in our bodies can be measured by testing saliva, giving us a good indication of how stressed we are.

α-amylase is an enzyme found in both saliva and pancreatic juice, which breaks down starches in our food. It has been found that the concentration of α-amylase in our saliva reflects the level of activity in the sympathetic nervous system.

Both these substances are stress indicators and can be measured in both laboratory and field experiments by testing saliva. However, we have to take care when collecting the data. Cortisol levels change throughout the day, so in order to compare results, we have to take measurements at the same time each day. In addition, the device that measures levels of α-amylase uses an enzyme reaction, so when the temperature is lower, so is the reading. For this reason, we have to collect data at the same temperature.

MEASURING
IMMUNE ACTIVITY

Natural killer (NK) cells are a type of lymphocyte, white blood cells that play a vital role in our immune systems. They form the front line in the body's defence system, guarding against tumours and attacking infections. We know that the level of activity of these cells is closely related to the level of stress or relaxation in our bodies. As stress increases, the activity of these cells decreases, reducing our ability to fight infection and tumour cells.

NK cells are a good indicator when it comes to clarifying how nature therapy improves immune function in subjects whose immunity has decreased due to stress. The level of NK cells is measured with a blood test, so this test isn't quite as easy to perform when subjects are walking in a forest or a city.

FIELD AND LABORATORY EXPERIMENTS

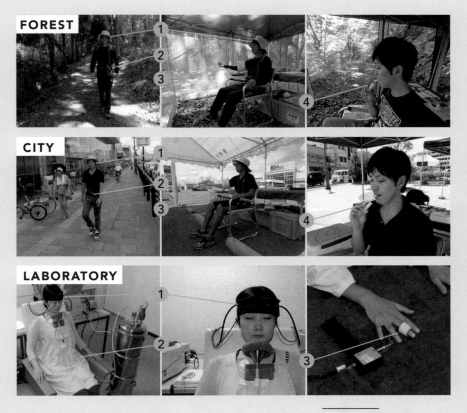

1. Sensors measuring prefrontal brain activity

2. Device to measure heart rate and HRV, recording autonomic nervous activity

3. Blood pressure measurement

4. Saliva sampling to measure level of cortisol

RESEARCH IN ACTION

The photographs above show data being collected in a laboratory and in the field, in both a city and a forest setting. The devices we use in the field are chosen because they are practical and can be used, in many cases, while the subject is moving around.

Research into forest therapy

Between 2005 and 2017, we ran a joint research programme between the Center for Environment, Health and Field Sciences, Chiba University and the Forestry and Forest Products Research Institute to study the physiological and psychological effects of forest therapy.

First we took an overview of the research that had already been done around the world, but we didn't find anything relating to the physiological effects provided by forests. So we started to think how to design our experiments from scratch. I remember spending two months constantly thinking about how to design the experiments, and running imaginary experiments in my head.

We first had to decide where to run the experiments. In order to clarify the effects of *shinrin-yoku*, we would need to compare our results with something. Therefore, we decided to compare *shinrin-yoku* to the urban environment in which we live.

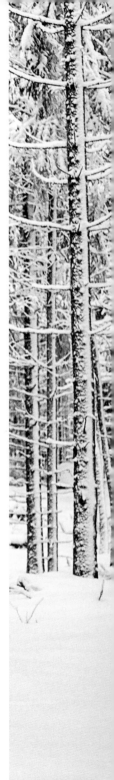

EXPERIMENT 1:
DOES FOREST THERAPY WORK?

We conducted our experiments in 63 forests across Japan, from Okinawa to Hokkaido, and ran the same set of experiments in urban areas nearby to act as a control.

Japan is a long, thin country running from north to south, and has distinctive forests that vary from region to region. For this reason, the selection of locations for our experiments was extremely important. We chose a forest that was typical of each region, and inspected the area twice before the experiments to choose specific locations. The experiments in each area involved 20 researchers and 12 subjects, and the two different parts (forest and urban) were designed to take place simultaneously, so preparation was the key to success.

Who we tested

We tested 12 Japanese university students in each region, all non-smokers and none taking any medication. In total, there were 756 subjects: 684 men and 72 women. In each region, we split the group in half: on the first day, six subjects were sent to a forest area, and the others to an urban area. On the second day, each group was sent to the other area as a cross-check.

What we tested

The subjects each spent 15 minutes walking in the morning, and 15 minutes just sitting and viewing in the afternoon. During the experiments, we measured the following:

· Autonomic nervous activity using heart rate variability (see page 134)

· Pulse rate (see page 134)

· Blood pressure (see page 134). Blood pressure readings have two numbers, for example 120/80. The top number is *systolic* blood pressure (the highest pressure when your heart beats and pushes the blood round your body), while the bottom one is *diastolic* blood pressure (the lowest pressure when your heart relaxes between beats)

· The stress marker cortisol in the subjects' saliva (see page 137)

· How the subjects felt, by asking them a series of questions

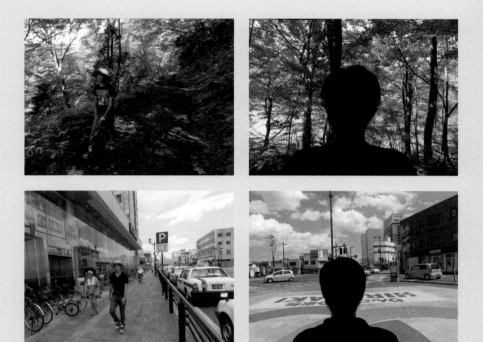

The subjects were asked to walk slowly through the forest or urban environment in the morning (left), then just sit and look at the view in the afternoon (right), before repeating the experiment in the other environment the next day.

The schedule

We gathered the 12 subjects together the day before the experiments and took them to have a look at both the forest and urban locations. When people do something for the first time, the novelty can cause unexpected physiological changes, so we showed them the locations before the actual experiments and explained the schedule. They then went to a hotel, all ate the same meal and stayed overnight in their rooms.

On the first day of experiments, the subjects were woken at 6am and, before breakfast, we took measurements to assess their stress levels. Next, they travelled by bus for between one and two hours to a waiting room in a forest or urban area (we arranged the travel time to be the same for both groups). On the second day, the forest group went to the urban area and vice versa, to make sure the results weren't affected by the order of the experiments. People can react differently to the same event depending on whether they are experiencing it for the first time or the second time. For example, if we tested all our subjects in the forest first and the urban environment second, we wouldn't know whether any differences in their reactions were due to being in the forest itself, or simply taking part in the experiments for the first time.

Also, we know that physiological indicators vary at different times of day, so we had to be aware of this when planning when to take the measurements, making sure each subject underwent the experiments in the same order and at the same time of day.

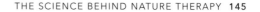

The walking experiments took place in the morning for 15 minutes per person, the subjects walking at the same speed in both forest and urban areas so that the amount of exercise would be the same. We took pulse rate, blood pressure and salivary cortisol concentration measurements before and after walking. During the walking, we measured the subjects' heart rate variability (to show their sympathetic and parasympathetic nerve activity) at one-minute intervals. In the afternoon, the 15-minute seated viewing experiments followed the same procedure as the walking experiments.

After the experiments, the subjects returned to their hotel, all ate the same dinner, then went to bed at an early hour. We prepared all the meals eaten during the experiments and the subjects were not allowed any other food or drink. When it rained, we cancelled that day's experiments and extended the session.

All these details meant that if we found any differences between our results in the forest and those in the urban areas, we could be confident that they were caused by differences between the two environments.

The results

Through these experiments, we were able to show[8-30] that during their time in the forest, subjects experienced:

· A decrease in sympathetic nerve activity (known to increase during times of stress)

· An increase in parasympathetic nerve activity (known to increase during relaxation)

· A decrease in blood pressure

· A decrease in pulse rate

· A decrease in the concentration of the stress hormone cortisol

It became clear that during forest therapy, the body experiences physiological relaxation.

The information on the questionnaires about how the subjects were feeling correlated well with the results of the physiological evaluation. The subjects reported that they felt:

· An increased feeling of comfort

· An increased feeling of calm

· An increase in feeling refreshed

· An improvement in their emotional state

· A reduction in anxiety

Results from seated viewing vs walking experiments

The table below shows the results from 24 of our locations, comparing the measurements taken during the seated viewing experiments with those taken during the forest walking experiments.[10] The values shown are the differences between the forest activity and the same activity performed in an urban setting.

	Seated forest viewing	Forest walking
Cortisol concentration (from saliva)	↓ 13.4%	↓ 15.8%
Pulse rate	↓ 6.0%	↓ 3.9%
Systolic blood pressure	↓ 1.7%	↓ 1.9%
Diastolic blood pressure	↓ 1.6%	↓ 2.1%
Parasympathetic nerve activity	↑ 56.0%	↑ 102.0%
Sympathetic nerve activity	↓ 18.0%	↓ 19.4%

The results of these experiments show that the body experiences physiological relaxation when we spend time in a forest.

EXPERIMENT 2: MEASURING BRAIN ACTIVITY

We also conducted experiments to measure brain activity using a time-resolved version of near-infrared spectroscopy[9] (see page 132). The set-up for the experiments was the same as those described above.

Who we tested

We tested 12 male subjects, average age 22.8 years.

What we tested

As before, the subjects stayed in individual hotel rooms from the day before the experiments to their finish, and ate the same meals. We measured their prefrontal brain activity five times each day. The first measurement was taken before breakfast at the hotel. Following that, the subjects were split into two groups, one travelling to the forest and one to an urban area. The second and third measurements took place before and after a 20-minute walk. The fourth and fifth measurements took place before and after 20 minutes of seated viewing.

The results

We found that during both walking and seated
viewing in the forest, the subjects' brain activity
reduced, indicating a state of physiological
relaxation. This experiment, conducted in 2007,
was the first in the world to demonstrate a calming
of prefrontal brain activity during forest therapy.

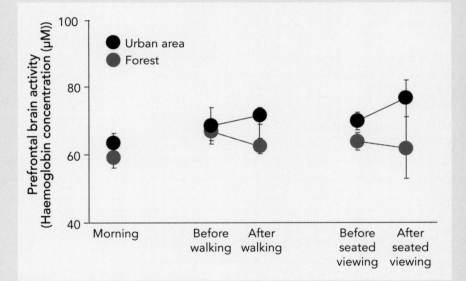

If we compare the results of
these experiments it is clear
that the body experiences
physiological relaxation
(indicated by a decrease
in brain activity) when we
spend time in a forest.

EXPERIMENT 3: THE EFFECTS OF FOREST THERAPY ON MEN WITH HIGH BLOOD PRESSURE

Next we wanted to test what effect a forest therapy session would have on a group of male subjects who had raised blood pressure.[15] We conducted the experiment in a forest in Agematsu, Nagano Prefecture from 10:30am to 3:05pm.

Who we tested

These experiments involved a group of nine men with existing high blood pressure, average age 56 years.

What we tested

We took the following measurements at the end of the forest therapy session:

· Blood pressure
· The concentration of the stress hormone adrenaline in the subjects' urine (which increases in conditions of stress)
· The concentration of the stress hormone cortisol in the subjects' blood (which increases in conditions of stress)

We also took readings at the same time of day on the day before the experiment so we could compare the results taken after the therapy with the subjects' usual results.

The results

We were able to show that after the forest therapy session:

· The subjects' systolic blood pressure dropped from 140.1 mmHg to 123.9 mmHg, while diastolic blood pressure dropped from 84.4 mmHg to 76.6 mmHg
· Adrenaline concentration levels fell
· Cortisol concentration levels fell

From these results, we were able to say that a forest therapy session lasting a few hours offered physiological relaxation effects to male subjects with high blood pressure.

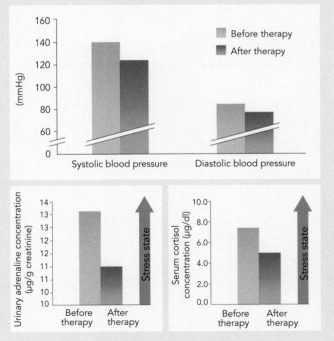

These graphs show a fall in (top) blood pressure, (bottom left) adrenaline levels and (bottom right) cortisol levels in men with high blood pressure after a forest therapy session.

EXPERIMENT 4:
THE EFFECTS OF FOREST THERAPY
ON OFFICE WORKERS

We also investigated the effects of a forest therapy session on the blood pressure of a group of office workers, some of whom were known to have high blood pressure. The experiment took place near the town of Chizu, Tottori Prefecture from 9am to 3:30pm.[13]

Who we tested

The subjects were 26 office workers, average age 35.7 years.

What we tested

We measured the subjects' systolic and diastolic blood pressure three times a day (before breakfast, lunch and dinner), on four different days:

· Three days before the forest therapy (at home or at work)
· On the day of the forest therapy
· Three days after the forest therapy
· Five days after the forest therapy

The results

Systolic and diastolic blood pressure went down significantly during the forest therapy session, relative to the value from three days before. This decrease was maintained three and five days after the forest therapy programme.

We then focused on nine subjects whose systolic blood pressure was above 120mmHg. Their average systolic blood pressure readings before dinner were 133.8mmHg three days before forest therapy. These decreased to 116.6mmHg during the forest therapy, to 126.4mmHg three days after, and to 124.0mmHg five days after the forest therapy. In other words, for measurements taken after the subjects had finished a day's work and before they ate dinner, lower blood pressure persisted for five days after forest therapy, even in the workplace. Diastolic blood pressure readings showed a similar tendency.

The graphs below show that blood pressure goes down when we spend time in a forest and this effect is maintained for several days afterwards.

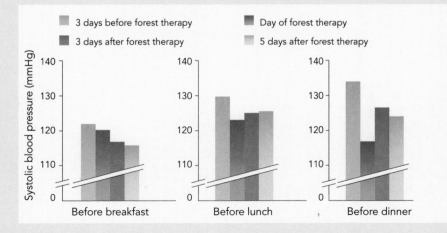

A FOREST THERAPY SESSION
FOR OFFICE WORKERS

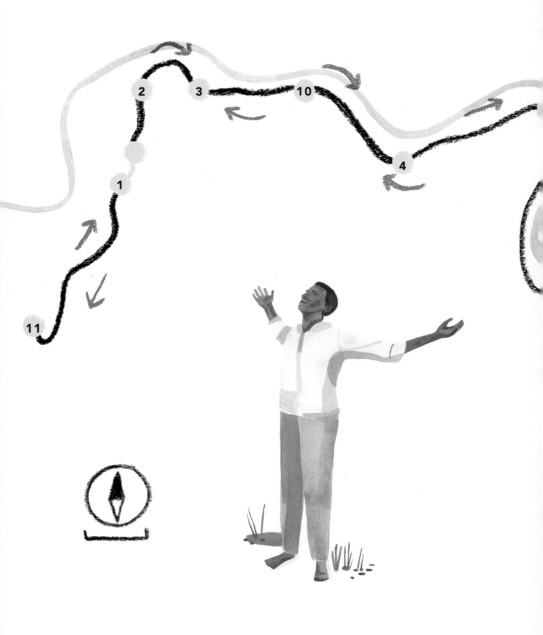

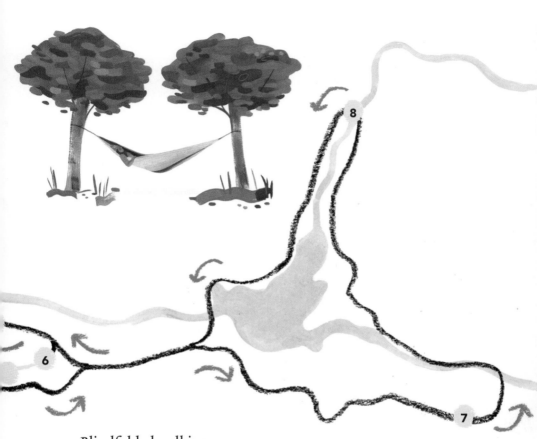

1. Blindfolded walking
2. Deep breathing
3. Viewing scenery
4. Washing away your cares
5. Sitting
6. Backward walking
7. Measurement before lunch
8. Meditation
9. Hammock
10. Deep breathing
11. Measurement after programme

This plan shows the route of the forest therapy session for office workers and the activities they experienced. The session lasted about 6½ hours.

EXPERIMENT 5:
THE EFFECTS OF FOREST
THERAPY ON MATURE WOMEN

Here we investigated the effects of a forest therapy session
on a group of mature women to see whether they would also
experience the same benefits. The therapy took place in a forest
in Agematsu, Nagano Prefecture from 10:30am to 3pm.[14]

Who we tested

This experiment involved a group of 17 mature women, ranging
from 40 to 73 years, average age 62.2 years.

What we tested

We took the following measurements at the end of the forest
therapy session:

· Blood pressure
· The concentration of the stress hormone cortisol in the
  subjects' saliva (which increases in conditions of stress)
· Pulse rate

We also took readings at the same time of day on the day before
the experiment so we could compare the results taken after the
therapy with the subjects' usual results.

The results

We found that the concentration of salivary cortisol (a typical stress hormone) had decreased by 26 per cent compared to the measurements taken the previous day.

The average pulse rate was also significantly lower after the subjects walked in a forest environment than on the day before forest therapy. Because the pulse rate is related to autonomic nervous system activity, the drop in pulse rate indicates a state of greater relaxation.

From these results, we can say that a forest therapy session of just a few hours provided physiological relaxation benefits to mature women.

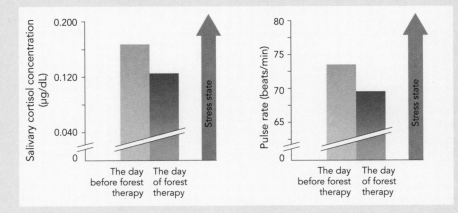

The cortisol levels and pulse rates of mature women decreased during forest therapy.

A FOREST THERAPY SESSION
FOR MATURE WOMEN

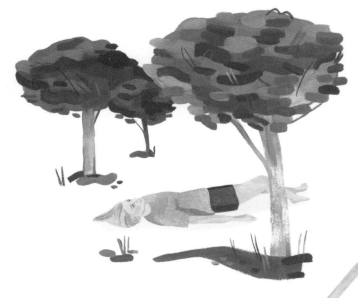

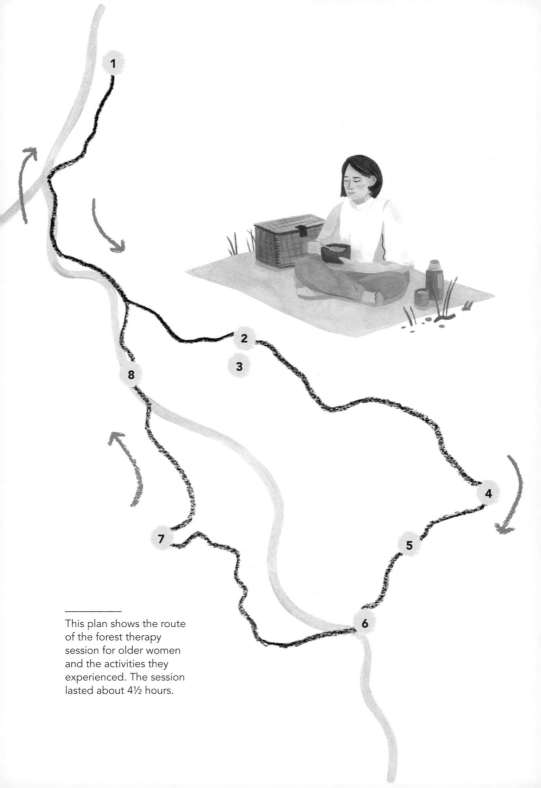

This plan shows the route of the forest therapy session for older women and the activities they experienced. The session lasted about 4½ hours.

Can forest therapy affect immune function?

As well as reducing stress levels in the body, forest therapy has been shown to improve immunity by increasing levels of natural killer (NK) cells. As we have seen, NK cells form a crucial part of the body's defence system, helping to fight infection and tumours (see page 138). Three studies by Dr Qing Li and his colleagues have demonstrated how forest therapy can have a beneficial effect on weakened immune function.

The subjects in the first study were 12 male office workers with weakened immune function, aged between 37 and 55 years. They participated in a three-day forest therapy course.[28] On Day 1 of the course, after a two-hour forest therapy walk, NK cell activity had increased by 1.25 times compared to measurements taken three days before the study. After forest therapy on Day 2, NK cell activity had increased by 1.5 times. This study confirmed the immunity-boosting effects of forest therapy on NK cell activity.

A similar experiment on female nurses also showed improvements in weakened NK cell activity.[29]

Li and his colleagues also studied the long-term effects of forest therapy on immune function.[29, 30]

Measurements were taken one week and one month after the subjects of the two experiments mentioned above returned to work. One week after the forest therapy, NK cell activity levels were still raised in both the male and female groups, and they were found to be still raised in the male group one month later.

To act as a control, the male group underwent the same programme in an urban setting and the results showed no improvement in NK cell activity.[30]

To recap

- Forest therapy improves weakened NK cell activity in male and female participants.

- These effects last for at least a week, and for the male participants lasted for one month.

- These improvements were not shown by walking in an urban environment.

Research into park therapy

Parks are valuable natural environments within our cities and most people have access to one. In fact, the local park is the only natural space available to many of us. Parks and other urban green spaces are becoming increasingly necessary in modern society.

Although most of us would recognize the park as a space where we feel relaxed, very little scientific research has been done to see whether this is in fact true. In this section I will examine whether parks can be as valuable as natural forests in offering the same physiological relaxation effects to stressed city-dwellers.[39–44]

EXPERIMENT 1: PARK VS URBAN WALK

To examine the possible benefits of simply taking a stroll in the park, we conducted a series of experiments in Shinjuku Gyoen, a famous park in Tokyo,[42] the most populous city in the world. We conducted the same experiments in the urban area around Shinjuku station to act as a control. The average atmospheric temperature was 29–30°C (84–86°F) and the humidity 66–67 per cent.

Who we tested

The subjects were 18 male Japanese university students who each spent 20 minutes walking in the park and in the urban area.

What we tested

While the subjects were walking, we measured their heart
rate variability (see page 134) and their pulse rate. We also asked
the subjects a series of questions about how they were feeling,
in particular about their levels of comfort, calm and accord
with nature.

The results

We found that, compared to walking in the urban area around
Shinjuku station, walking in Shinjuku Gyoen park resulted in:

· An increase in parasympathetic nerve activity (known to
  increase during relaxation)

· A lower pulse rate

· An increased feeling of comfort, calm and accord with nature

In other words, we showed that walking in Shinjuku Gyoen, an
urban park in the middle of a large city, does physiologically relax
the human body.

Research into other nature therapies

EXPERIMENT 1: ORNAMENTAL PLANTS

Most people would say that having ornamental plants in the house or workplace engenders a sense of wellbeing, but we wanted to investigate whether houseplants have the same relaxation effects as other natural stimuli, particularly on young people. We used three *Dracaena deremensis* plants, 55–60cm (21–24 inches) in height, spaced 8cm (3 inches) apart. Some subjects looked at the plants for 3 minutes, others looked at the same view without the plants.

Who we tested

We conducted our experiments on 85 high school students, 41 boys and 44 girls, average age 16.5 years.[57]

What we tested

While the subjects were viewing the plant (or not), we measured their heart rate variability and pulse rate to gauge levels of parasympathetic nerve activity (higher at times of relaxation) and sympathetic nerve activity (higher at times of stress).

After the experiment, the subjects were asked to rate how they were feeling using three different scales: "comfortable–uncomfortable", "relaxed–stressed" and "natural–artificial".

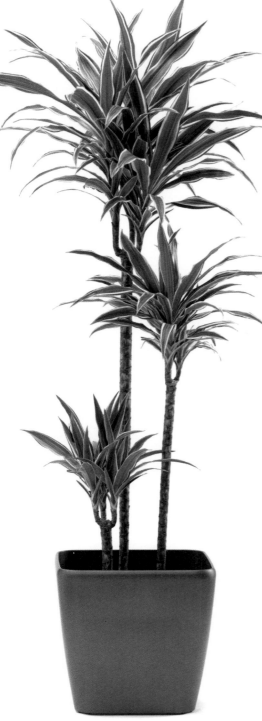

The results

The results indicated a 13.5 per cent increase in parasympathetic nerve activity and a 5.6 per cent suppression of sympathetic nerve activity while viewing the ornamental plants rather than the control. The subjects were also more likely to report that they felt more comfortable, relaxed and natural.

This means that ornamental plants do provide a physiological relaxation effect in young people and plant displays in high schools may be an effective way to relieve stress levels among students.

EXPERIMENT 2: BONSAI

Bonsai has been a popular art form in Japan for a very long time, and offers a way to bring nature into people's everyday lives. Bonsai is designed to mimic scenes from nature, and has recently become one of Japan's best-known cultural exports. Despite this, no one has studied the effects of the physiological reactions produced by bonsai. We wanted to know how simply viewing bonsai could affect stress levels in humans.

Who we tested

Our subjects were individuals who had suffered spinal cord injuries, which would have made forest therapy difficult. The subjects were 24 males (average age 49) with spinal cord injuries, who were able to operate their wheelchairs by themselves.[71]

What we tested

We asked the subjects to look at a group of eight hinoki trees planted together in a pot, or look at nothing, for 60 seconds. All subjects experienced both options, which were presented in a random order. During the experiment, we used near-infrared spectroscopy (see pages 132–3) to gauge activity levels in the brain, which reflect stress levels. We also measured heart rate variability (see page 134) to record activity in the parasympathetic and sympathetic nervous systems. The subjects were asked how they were feeling during the experiments.

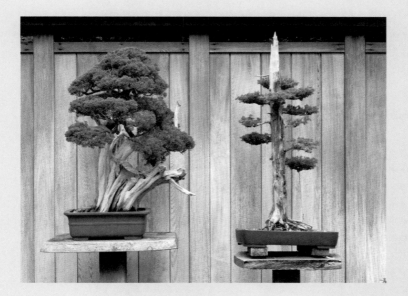

The results

The results showed that, compared to the control, viewing bonsai produced:

· A calming of prefrontal brain activity (oxygenated haemoglobin in the left prefrontal area)

· An increase in activity in the parasympathetic nervous system (which increases during times of relaxation)

· A decrease in activity in the sympathetic nervous system (which increases during times of stress)

· An increase in positive feelings

To sum up, viewing bonsai relaxed the subjects, both physiologically and psychologically. As depressive disorders are very common among people who have suffered spinal cord injuries, bonsai therapy might be a way to improve feelings of relaxation and wellbeing, and is something people can do themselves at home.

EXPERIMENT 3: FLOWER ARRANGEMENTS

Flower arrangements are an easy way to bring nature into our daily lives, whether in the home, office or public space. We know that cut flowers give us pleasure, but do they offer physical benefits too? We wanted to investigate whether flower arrangements could contribute to reducing the stresses of modern life by acting as a kind of preventative medicine. Could fresh flowers in the workplace help office workers who are experiencing high levels of stress?

Our experiments examined whether an arrangement of cut roses could relax the human body. To make sure our results weren't confused by the effects of scent from the flowers, we used unscented roses. Our arrangement consisted of 30 pink roses with 40cm (16-inch) stems, arranged in a tubular glass vase 20cm (8 inches) high and 12cm (5 inches) in diameter.

Who we tested

The experimental subjects were high-school pupils, female health professionals and office workers.[62–65]

What we tested

Each subject viewed the unscented flower arrangement in a special room from a distance of 37–40cm (15–16 inches) for four minutes, or viewed the same room without the flowers. We measured the subjects' heart rate variability and pulse rate to gauge the level of activity in their parasympathetic and sympathetic nervous systems. We also asked the subjects a series of questions to rate their level of comfort and relaxation.

The results

· We found that the high school students[62] experienced a 16.7 per cent rise in parasympathetic nerve activity and a 30.5 per cent drop in sympathetic nerve activity.

· The medical professionals[64] experienced a 33.1 per cent rise in parasympathetic nerve activity.

· The results from the office workers as a whole did not show such a marked effect, but when we analyzed the results from the 31 male office workers,[63] they showed a 21.1 per cent rise in parasympathetic nerve activity.

· The results from the same experiment conducted on another 114 subjects[65] showed a 15.1 per cent rise in parasympathetic nerve activity and a 16.3 per cent reduction in sympathetic nerve activity. These results are shown on the graph below.

As we know that activity in the parasympathetic nervous system increases during times of relaxation, while activity in the sympathetic nervous system increases during times of stress, we concluded from these experiments that simply looking at an arrangement of flowers increases relaxation and decreases stress.

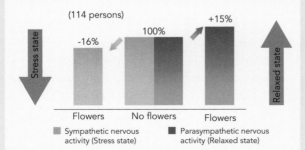

Viewing an arrangement of cut roses increased relaxation levels and decreased stress levels in the 114 participants.

EXPERIMENT 4: FLOWER SCENT

This experiment examined whether the scent of flowers had the same relaxing effect on the body as looking at flowers does. We wanted to find out whether essential oils extracted from flowers, which have been used for millenia, offer any physiological benefits. To find out, we asked subjects to breathe in the aroma of rose and orange essential oils.

Who we tested

We conducted our experiment on 20 female university students, average age 22.5 years.[68–70]

What we tested

Using a breathing device, subjects were exposed to 90 seconds of air impregnated with rose or orange essential oils. We had adjusted the aroma to a sensory strength between "very faint" and "weak". As a control, subjects wore the same device but inhaled air that had not been impregnated with scent. The three stimuli (rose, orange and plain air) were randomly presented to each subject.

During the experiment we used a time-resolved version of near-infrared spectroscopy (see pages 132–3) to measure the level of prefrontal brain activity in each subject, which reflects the subject's level of stress. We also asked subjects to rate how they were feeling during the experiment in a questionnaire.

The results

We found that, compared to plain air, inhaling the scent of rose or orange oil decreased prefrontal brain activity and, therefore, stress levels in the subjects. They were also more likely to report they felt comfortable, relaxed and natural.

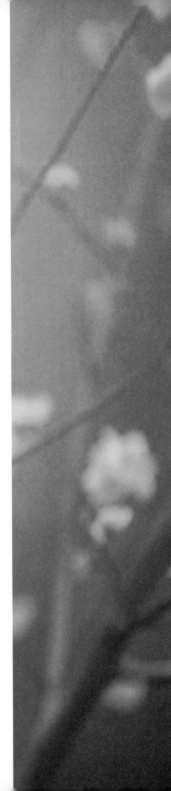

EXPERIMENT 5:
THE SCENT OF WOOD

Wood has a special meaning for Japanese people, and is closely linked to their daily lives in the form of furniture, artworks, small everyday items and even as a construction material to build houses.

Wood needs to be dried out to prevent warping before it can be used as a construction material, and these days much of it is dried artificially by heat processing. We know that heating can alter the substances found in wood, and those with a low boiling point can evaporate altogether. This changes the "natural" smell of wood. We decided to investigate the different physiological relaxation effects provided by naturally dried wood versus heat-treated wood.[52]

We asked our subjects to inhale the aroma of two different types of hinoki (*Chamaecyparis obtusa*) wood chips sourced from Kumamoto Prefecture. The naturally dried wood had been sawn then dried for 45 months, while the heat-treated wood had been dried rapidly using intense heat.

Who we tested

We tested 19 female university students, average age 22.5 years.

What we tested

The subjects were asked to inhale the two aromas for 90 seconds. We adjusted the strength of the aromas to a sensory strength of between "very faint" and "weak". We recorded the subjects' brain activity (the concentration of oxygenated haemoglobin in the left prefrontal area) as a measure of their level of relaxation.

The results

Our results confirmed a difference between the two materials: namely, that inhaling the aroma of naturally dried wood reduced the concentration of oxygenated haemoglobin in the brain, whereas there was no change after inhaling the aroma of heat-treated wood. This means that the smell of naturally dried wood calms prefrontal brain activity and relaxes the human body.

Using aroma compounds alone

We performed a similar experiment to determine the effects on the body of plant aroma compounds used on their own.[50, 51] We used α-pinene and limonene, two typical forest-derived compounds which are produced by trees such as cedar, pine and citrus. We found that after inhaling these compounds, subjects experienced the same physiological relaxation effects as when inhaling the aroma of naturally dried wood and reported feelings of relaxation and comfort.

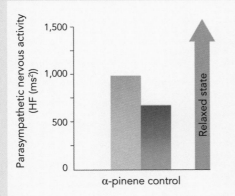

The graph shows that inhaling α-pinene, a plant-derived aroma compound, leads to increased activity in the parasympathetic nervous system, which is known to occur during times of relaxation.

"Trees are poems
that earth writes
upon the sky"

— KAHLIL GIBRAN

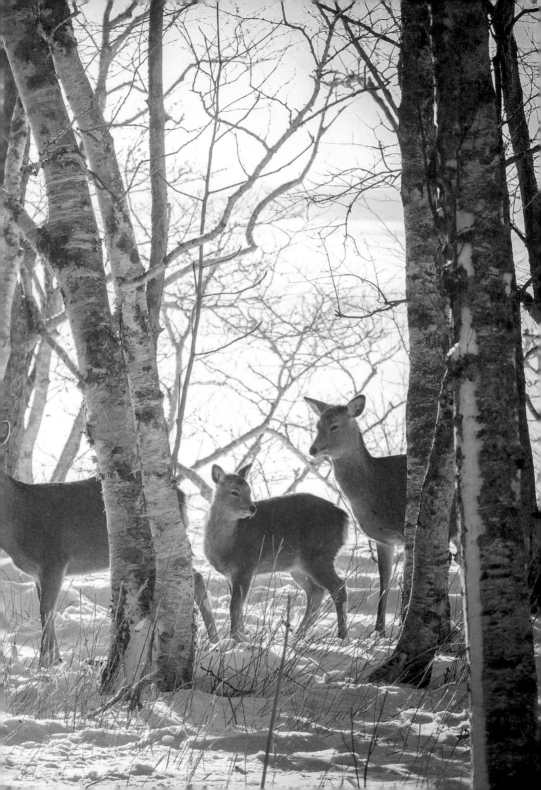

CHAPTER 6

The Future of Forest Therapy Research

森林セラピー研究のこれから

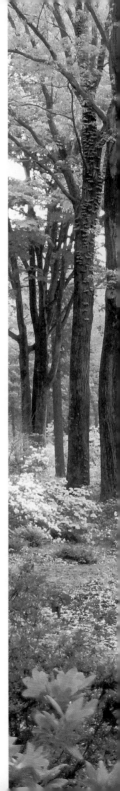

It is encouraging to see the practice of forest bathing growing in popularity around the world. The question at the heart of research into nature therapies such as forest therapy is how nature affects people. But right now, there are no academic institutions that teach about both nature and people together, either in Japan, Europe or the United States. It is possible to study forests, parks, timber and flowers, but not to combine these subjects with the study of human beings, who are affected by them. On the other hand, there is plenty of medical research being done on people, but not how they relate to nature.

In today's stressful society, there is global interest in how stimulation from nature can reduce stress and provide relaxation. Yet the current research system cannot produce researchers with the ability to cover all aspects of this subject. In Japan, there is a growing awareness of the harmful effect of rigid divisions between research fields. People are aware how important it is to merge research fields, yet somehow the situation doesn't improve.

The heads of both the Finnish Forest Research Institute and the Center for Health and Global Environment at the Harvard School of Public Health in the United States have asked me for

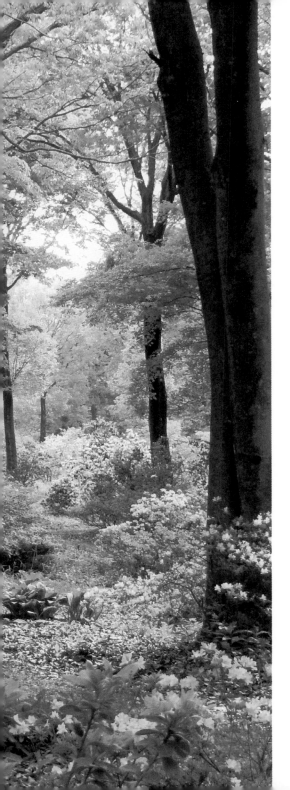

advice on how to merge their research with faculties of medicine. It is a key challenge to combine research into physical things such as a forests and timber with research into people. We are probably now in a transitional phase.

Presently, I am conducting my nature therapy research alongside my colleague, Assistant Professor Chorong Song, and Dr Harumi Ikei, a researcher at Japan's Forestry and Forest Products Research Institute. Dr Ikei studied my research as a high-school student and decided to become a forest therapy researcher. She applied to Chiba University, then got her PhD in my laboratory. Assistant Professor Chorong Song read a Korean translation of my research book and also decided to become a forest therapy researcher. She travelled to Japan and completed a masters course and doctorate before joining my laboratory as a researcher. They both continue to provide invaluable assistance in my current research.

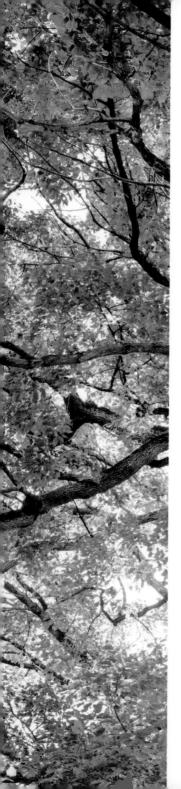

There is a history of close cooperation between Japan and South Korea in forest therapy research, and in 2015 a National Forest Healing Center was established in South Korea, with government funding to investigate the scientific effects of forest therapy, and to develop therapy programmes.

In the United States, two people have played a huge role in publicizing *shinrin-yoku* research around the world: Alan C Logan and Florence Williams. In their 2012 book,[4] *Your Brain on Nature*, Logan and Eva M Selhub write about the importance of nature in our urbanized and artificial society. Williams published her book *The Nature Fix*[73] in 2017, and I supplied an editorial for the Japanese translation the same year.

In the process of writing her book, Williams interviewed over 20 prominent nature therapy researchers from eight countries to determine why nature makes us happier, healthier and more creative. In my view, it is essential reading for anyone wishing to understand current global trends in forest therapy research.

Founded by M Amos Clifford, the Association of Nature and Forest Therapy Guides and Programs is leading the movement in the United States to integrate nature and other forest therapies into healthcare, education and land management so that, at some point in the future, healthcare providers may send patients to certified forest therapy guides for treatment, and forest therapy is accepted as a valuable treatment in the same way as mindfulness meditation is.

It is my belief that, in the modern world, forest therapy and other nature therapies are the most practical way to reduce our stress levels and increase relaxation. At the end of the day, our bodies are adapted to nature. I believe that nature can be a considerable help in reducing the strain on healthcare services all over the world. With my research, I hope to continue contributing to the popularization of nature therapy.

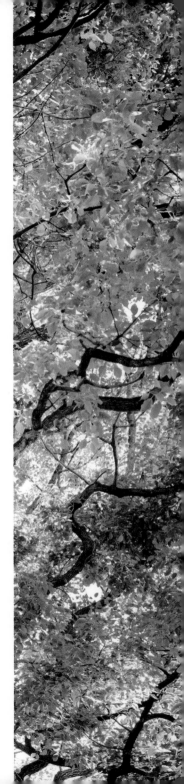

"The wonder is that we can see these trees and not wonder more"

— RALPH WALDO EMERSON

FOREST THERAPY ORGANIZATIONS

The Association of Nature & Forest Therapy Guides & Programs

Based in the United States, this organization aims to integrate nature and forest therapies into health care, education and land management systems. It trains and certifies forest therapy guides from all over the world A page on their website gives details of certified guides around the world.

www.natureandforesttherapy.org

Australasian Nature & Forest Therapy Alliance

Based in Melbourne, Australia, this organization aims to promote nature and forest therapy in Australia, Asia and internationally, and to support nature and forest therapists in their work.

anfta.org

Forest Holidays, UK

Supported and part-owned by the Forestry Commission, this company offers wood cabins to holidaymakers in some of Britain's forests. Forest therapy sessions are available at two of the sites, Blackwood Forest in Hampshire and Thorpe Forest in Norfolk.

www.forestholidays.co.uk

Forest Therapy Scotland

A company offering forest therapy sessions across the country.

forest-therapy-scotland.com

Forest Therapy Society, Japan

An organization created to support the practice of forest therapy and certify Forest Therapy Bases and Forest Therapy Roads across Japan. The website is in Japanese.

www.fo-society.jp/therapy

Korea Forest Service

Set up to protect and nurture forests all over South Korea, and promote recreation and forest activities. There is a network of designated stations for forest bathing (known as *salim yok*).

english.forest.go.kr

REFERENCES

1 *Shinrin-yoku* (forest bathing) plan by Forest Agency, The Asahi Shimbun, July 29, 1982 (in Japanese)

2 Changes in salivary cortisol concentration and psychological indicator by *shinrin-yoku* (forest bathing), Japanese Journal of Biometeorology, 27 (Suppl.), 1990 (in Japanese)

3 TIME The healing power of nature, July 25, 2016

4 E.M. Selhub and A.C. Logan, *Your Brain On Nature*, John Wiley & Sons, 2013

5 Brunet, M. et al. A new hominid from the Upper Miocene of Chad, Central Africa. Nature 418, 141–151, 2002

6 C. Song, H. Ikei and Y. Miyazaki. Physiological effects of nature therapy: A review of the research in Japan. Int J Environ Res Public Health 13(8) 781, 2016

7 Y. Miyazaki, *The Science of Nature Therapy*, Asakura Publishing, 2016 (in Japanese)

8 C. Song, H. Ikei and Y. Miyazaki. Elucidation of a physiological adjustment effect in a forest environment: a pilot study. Int J Environ Res Public Health 12 4247–4255, 2015

9 B.J. Park, Y. Miyazaki et al. Physiological effects of *shinrin-yoku* (taking in the atmosphere of the forest) using salivary cortisol and cerebral activity as indicators. Journal of Physiological Anthropology 26(2): 123–128, 2007

10 B.J. Park, Y. Miyazaki et al. The physiological effects of *shinrin-yoku* (taking in the forest atmosphere or forest bathing): evidence from field experiments in 24 forests across Japan. Environmental Health and Preventive Medicine 15(1): 18–26, 2010

11 Y. Ohe, Y. Miyazaki et al. Evaluating the relaxation effects of emerging forest-therapy tourism: A multidisciplinary approach. Tourism Manage 62 322–334, 2017

12 C. Song, Y. Miyazaki et al. Effects of viewing forest landscape on middle-aged hypertensive men. Urban For Urban Gree 21 247–252, 2017

13 C. Song, H. Ikei and Y. Miyazaki. Sustained effects of a forest therapy program on the blood pressure of office workers. Urban For Urban Gree 27 246–252, 2017

14 H. Ochiai, Y. Miyazaki et al. Physiological and psychological effects of a forest therapy program on middle-aged females. Int J Environ Res Public Health 12(12) 15222–15232, 2015

15 H. Ochiai, Y. Miyazaki et al. Physiological and psychological effects of forest therapy on middle-aged males with high–normal blood pressure. Int J Environ Res Public Health 12 2532–2542, 2015

16 C. Song, Y. Miyazaki et al. Effect of forest walking on autonomic nervous system activity in middle-aged hypertensive individuals. Int J Environ Res Public Health 12 2687–2699, 2015

17 H. Kobayashi, Y. Miyazaki et al. Population-based study on the effect of a forest environment on salivary cortisol concentration. Int J Environ Res Public Health 14(8) 931, 2017

18 H. Kobayashi, Y. Miyazaki et al. Analysis of individual variations in autonomic responses to urban and forest environments. Evid Based Complement Alternat Med 671094, 2015

19 J. Lee, Y. Miyazaki et al. Acute effects of exposure to traditional rural environment on urban dwellers: a crossover field study in terraced farmland. Int J Environ Res Public Health 12 1874–1893, 2015

20 J. Lee, Y. Miyazaki et al. Influence of forest therapy on cardiovascular relaxation in young adults. Evid Based Complement Alternat Med 834360, 2014

21 Y. Tsunetsugu, Y. Miyazaki et al. Physiological and psychological effects of viewing urban forest landscapes assessed by multiple measurements. Landscape Urban Plan 113 90–93, 2013

22 Y. Tsunetsugu, Y. Miyazaki et al. Physiological effects of *shinrin-yoku* (taking in the atmosphere of the forest) in an old-growth broadleaf forest in Yamagata Prefecture, Japan. J Physiol Anthropol, 26(2), 135–142, 2007

23 J. Lee, Y. Miyazaki et al. Restorative effects of viewing real forest landscapes, based on a comparison with urban landscapes, Scand J Forest Res, 24(3), 227–234, 2009

24 B.J. Park, Y. Miyazaki et al. Physiological effects of forest recreation in a young conifer forest in Hinokage town, Japan. Silva Fenn, 43(2), 291–301, 2009

25 J. Lee, Y. Miyazaki et al. Effect of forest bathing on physiological and psychological responses in young Japanese male subjects, Public Health, 125(2), 93–100, 2011

26 C. Song, Y. Miyazaki et al. Individual differences in the physiological effects of forest therapy based

on Type A and Type B behavior patterns. J Physiol Anthropol 32(14) doi: 10.1186/1880–6805–32–14, 2013

27 Y. Tsunetsugu, Y. Miyazaki et al. Trends in research related to *shinrin-yoku* (taking in the forest atmosphere or forest bathing) in Japan. Environ Health Prev Med 15(1): 27–37, 2010

28 Q. Li, Y. Miyazaki et al. Forest bathing enhances human natural killer activity and expression of anti-cancer proteins. Int J Immunopathol Pharmacol 20(S2) 3–8, 2007

29 Q. Li, Y. Miyazaki et al. A forest bathing trip increases human natural killer activity and expression of anti-cancer proteins in female subjects. J Biol Regul Homeost Agents 22(1) 45–55, 2008

30 Q. Li, Y. Miyazaki et al. Visiting a forest, but not a city, increases human natural killer activity and expression of anti-cancer proteins. Int J Immunopathol Pharmacol 21(1) 117–127, 2008

31 M. Sato, The story of life sciences, Japanese Standards Association 1994 (in Japanese)

32 M.A. O'Grady and L. Meinecke, Journal of Societal and Cultural Research 1(1) 1–25, 2015

33 R.S. Ulrich, View through a window may influence recovery from surgery, Science 224, 4647, 420–421, 1984

34 M. Inui, *Flexible environmental theory*, Kaimeisya Corporation, 1988 (in Japanese)

35 I. Kurita, *A Flower Journey*. Iwanami Shoten Publishers, 2001 (in Japanese)

36 M. Watanabe, The concept of nature in Japanese culture, Science 183 (4122) 279–282, 1974

37 M. Watanabe, *The view of nature in Japanese*. Ed. S. Ito, Kawade Shobo Shinsha 1995 (in Japanese)

38 H. Morinaga, *Shizen* (Nature) (1) 52–58, 1976 (in Japanese)

39 C. Song, Y. Miyazaki et al. Physiological and psychological effects of a walk in urban parks in fall. Int J Environ Res Public Health 12(11) 14216–14228, 2015

40 C. Song, Y. Miyazaki et al. Physiological and psychological responses of young males during spring-time walks in urban parks. J Physiol Anthropol 33(8), 2014

41 C. Song, Y. Miyazaki et al. Physiological and psychological effects of walking on young males in urban parks in winter. J Physiol Anthropol 32(18), 2013

42 N. Matsuba, Y. Miyazaki et al. Physiological effects of walking in Shinjuku Gyoen: A large-scale urban green area, Jpn J Physiol Anthropol, 16(3): 133–139, 2011 (in Japanese with English abstract)

43 M. Igarashi, Y. Miyazaki et al. Physiological and psychological effects of viewing a kiwifruit (*Actinidia deliciosa* 'Hayward') orchard landscape in summer in Japan. Int J Environ Res Public Health 12(6): 6657–6668, 2015

44 K. Matsunaga, Y. Miyazaki et al. Physiologically relaxing effect of a hospital rooftop forest on older women requiring care. J Am Geriatr Soc 59(11) 2162–2163, 2011

45 Y. Miyazaki et al. Changes in mood by inhalation of essential oils in humans II. Effect of essential oils on blood pressure, heart rate, R–R intervals, performance, sensory evaluation and POMS. Mokuzai Gakkaishi 38:909–913, 1992 (in Japanese with English abstract)

46 H. Ikei, C. Song and Y. Miyazaki. Physiological effects of wood on humans: A review. J Wood Sci 63(1) 1–23, 2017

47 H. Ikei, C. Song and Y. Miyazaki. Physiological effects of touching hinoki cypress (*Chamaecyparis obtusa*). J Wood Sci doi: 10.1007/s10086–017–1691–7, 2018

48 H. Ikei, C. Song and Y. Miyazaki. Physiological effects of touching wood. Int J Environ Res Public Health 14(7) 801, 2017

49 H. Ikei, C. Song and Y. Miyazaki. Physiological effects of touching coated wood. Int J Environ Res Public Health 14(7) 773, 2017

50 H. Ikei, C. Song and Y. Miyazaki. Effects of olfactory stimulation by α-pinene on autonomic nervous activity. J Wood Sci 62(6) 568–572, 2016

51 D. Joung, Y. Miyazaki et al. Physiological and psychological effects of olfactory stimulation with D-limonene. Adv Hortic Sci 28(2) 90–94, 2014

52 H. Ikei, Y. Miyazaki et al. Comparison of the effects of olfactory stimulation by air-dried and high temperature-dried wood chips of hinoki cypress (*Chamaecyparis obtusa*) on prefrontal cortex activity. J Wood Sci 61 537–540, 2015

53 H. Ikei, C. Song and Y. Miyazaki. Physiological effect of olfactory stimulation by hinoki cypress (*Chamaecyparis obtusa*) leaf oil. J Physiol Anthropol 34(44), 2015

54 Q. Li, Y. Miyazaki et al. Effect of phytoncide from trees on human natural killer cell function. Int J Immunopathol Pharmacol 22(4) 951–959, 2009

55 M. Igarashi, Y. Miyazaki et al. Physiological and psychological effects on high school students of viewing real and artificial pansies. Int J Environ Res Public Health 12 2521–2531, 2015

56 M. Igarashi, Y. Miyazaki et al. Effect of stimulation by foliage plant display images on prefrontal cortex activity: A comparison with stimulation using actual foliage plants. J Neuroimaging 25 127–130, 2015

57 H. Ikei, Y. Miyazaki et al. Physiological and psychological relaxing effects of visual stimulation with foliage plants in high school students. Adv Hortic Sci 28(2) 111–116, 2014

58 S.A. Park, Y. Miyazaki et al. Comparison of physiological and psychological relaxation using measurements of heart rate variability, prefrontal cortex activity, and subjective indexes after completing tasks with and without foliage plants. Int J Environ Res Public Health 14(9)1087, 2017

59 S.A. Park, Y. Miyazaki et al. Foliage plants cause physiological and psychological relaxation, as evidenced by measurements of prefrontal cortex activity and profile of mood states. HortScience 51(10) 1308–1312, 2016

60 M.S. Lee, Y. Miyazaki et al. Interaction with indoor plants may reduce psychological and physiological stress by suppressing autonomic nervous system activity in young adults: a randomized crossover study. J Physiol Anthropol 34(21), 2015

61 M. Igarashi, Y. Miyazaki et al. Effects of stimulation by three-dimensional natural images on prefrontal cortex and autonomic nerve activity: a comparison with stimulation using two-dimensional images. Cogn Process 15(4) 551–556, 2014

62 H. Ikei, Y. Miyazaki et al. Physiological relaxation of viewing rose flowers in high school students. Jpn J Physiol Anthropol, 18(3): 97–103, 2013 (in Japanese with English abstract)

63 H. Ikei, Y. Miyazaki et al. The physiological and psychological relaxing effects of viewing rose flowers in office workers. J Physiol Anthropol, 33(6), 2014

64 M. Komatsu, Y. Miyazaki et al. The physiological and psychological relaxing effects of viewing rose flowers in medical staff. Jpn J Physiol Anthropol, 18(1): 1–7, 2014 (in Japanese with English abstract)

65 H. Ikei, Y. Miyazaki et al. Physiological relaxation of viewing roses – from the results of 114 subjects. Jap J Physiol Anthropol, 17(2): 150–151, 2012 (in Japanese)

66 C. Song, Y. Miyazaki et al. Physiological effects of viewing fresh red roses. Complement Ther Med 35: 78–84, 2017

67 M.S. Lee, Y. Miyazaki et al. Physiological relaxation induced by horticultural activity: transplanting work using flowering plants. J Physiol Anthropol 32(15), 2013

68 M. Igarashi, Y. Miyazaki et al. Effects of olfactory stimulation with rose and orange oil on prefrontal cortex activity. Complement Ther Med 22(6) 1027–1031, 2014

69 M. Igarashi, Y. Miyazaki et al. Effect of olfactory stimulation by fresh rose flowers on autonomic nervous activity. J Altern Complement Med 20(9) 727–731, 2014

70 B.J. Park, Y. Miyazaki et al. Physiological effects of orange essential oil inhalation in humans. Adv Hortic Sci 28(4) 225–230, 2014

71 H. Ochiai, Y. Miyazaki et al. Effects of visual stimulation with bonsai trees on adult male patients with spinal cord injury. Int J Environ Res Public Health 14(9)1017, 2017

72 M. Igarashi, Y. Miyazaki et al. Effects of olfactory stimulation with perilla essential oil on prefrontal cortex activity. J Altern Complement Med 20(7) 545–549, 2014.

73 F. Williams *The Nature Fix*. W W Norton & Co Inc., 2017

INDEX

PICTURE CREDITS

ACKNOWLEDGEMENTS

Dr Juyoung Lee helped me write the section on forest therapy in South Korea.

The section on forest therapy in the United States was written with the kind cooperation of Megumi Mizutani, a US-Japan cultural consultant based in Sebastopol, California.

I am grateful to Kate Adams for her contribution to pages 8–9, 30–3, 49, 52, 64 (top), 78–93, 100–2, 106 (bottom), 108–9 and 160–1.

I am grateful to Joanna Smith for her contribution to pages 35, 55–6, 98–9, 104–6 (top) and 110–22.

I would like to thank Dr Harumi Ikei for her editorial assistance.